I WILL

A MEMOIR OF STROKE, RENEWAL AND THE POWER OF SONG

Jenny Sheldon

with Sharon Dean

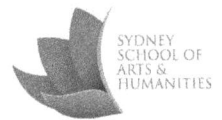

First edition: Sydney, 2018.
Publisher: Sydney School of Arts & Humanities
15-17 Argyle Place NSW 2000 Australia
www.ssoa.com.au

I WILL
ISBN: 978-0-648321613 (print)
       978-0-648321620 (ebook)

Copyright ©Jenny Sheldon, 2018. First published 2018.
All rights reserved. Without limiting the rights under copyright reserved above, no part of this publication may be reproduced, stored in or introduced into a retrieval system, or transmitted, in any form or by any means (electronic, mechanical, photocopying, recording or otherwise), without the prior written permission of both the copyright owner and the publisher.

What follows is a true story. Most dates, place names and events in this memoir are factual. However, in accordance with the wishes of certain participants, some names of people and places have been changed in order to protect privacy.
Cover design and Formatting Ferdinando Manzo
Typeset Times New Roman
Printed and bound by Lightning Source, 2018.

National Library of Australia Cataloguing-in-Publication data:
Sheldon, Jenny/Dean, Sharon, authors.
I WILL – Sheldon, Jenny/Dean, Sharon
ISBN 978-0-648321613 (print book)

Dedication

To my brother Mark
who was committed to the improvement of indigenous health
in Australia

Acknowledgements

My thanks to Bronwyn Green for not letting me take myself too seriously, and Denise Gerards and Jane Eliott, true friends – I appreciate that you all stood by me. Also to Deborah Martin-Smith for believing in me, Pippa Crane for believing I could write this book, and Karen Riley for the invaluable help she has given me. I am grateful to Karen Thompson, Laurie Abela, a special friend, and choir mates, Helen Spencer, Kathleen Mills, Helen Flanagan, and Josie and Colin Nicholson. Also Margaret Murphy from TAFE, and Dr John Watts and Dr Fiona Wagner for their health care.

Many thanks to all my friends who are too numerous to mention. You have enriched my life.

I would also like to thank Christine Williams from Sydney School of Arts & Humanities which is publishing this book. She is an inspiration to me and has become my friend. Thank you! My thanks too to Ferdinando Manzo from the School for his design and formatting skills.

I am especially grateful to Sharon Dean who went on a

'journey of my life' with me. It brought painful memories at times but she was able to make sense of it for me. I sang in the Northern Rivers Choir with her, and I never imagined she would help me tell my story. Sharon is so talented in having crafted the story. Thank you, Sharon!

And most of all, thanks to my family, the Sheldons. First to my mother, Winsome Gae, and my late father, Bruce Henry Gilbert. They have been my champions. Then thanks to my brother, John Henry Gilbert, and his partner Kirsty Gowan and their children, Jack, Riley and Caitlin. This book is for you all.

Special gratitude in memory of my late grandfather, Mervyn Lesley Gilbert, and my grandmother, Margaret – better known as Bamps and Maime. During his life Bamps, a musician, often quoted the following passage from an unknown source:

This is the luxury of music
It touches all the keys of memory
And stirs all the hidden streams
Of joy and of sorrow.
I love it for what it makes me forget
And for what it makes me remember.

Finally, a note for my late brother, Mark Lesley Gilbert: the Beatles still reign but I prefer ABBA.

CONTENTS

Prologue	13
PART 1	17
PART 2	40
PART 3	106
PART 4	127
EPILOGUE	160

PROLOGUE

It's my first night in rehab and my parents are helping me settle in. They wheel me into the dining room in a regency chair, and as I wait for my dinner we watch the news. On the screen are images of huge waves crashing right over the top of an enormous red ship. A reporter says the ship is a coal bulk carrier called the Pasha Bulker. Apparently, during a storm on June 8 of this year, which is 2007, the forty-thousand-tonne vessel had run aground at Nobby's Beach in Newcastle.

Mum mentions that I had my stroke that same day. I'm desperate to know what the date is now but can't ask. Since the stroke, I can say little more than, 'Yes', 'No', 'I don't think so'. But the newsreader gives me my answer! 'And that wraps up our program,' she says, 'for this Monday June 18.'

My brain is foggy but I do the maths. Is it really ten days since my stroke? A few hours ago I was transferred from Lismore Base Hospital to this rehabilitation unit in the seaside town of Ballina. Was I in hospital all that time?

A trolley with food arrives but I stare past it. In my mind I can still see the stranded ship. The weight of my despair grows heavier. The Pasha Bulker was grounded by a storm and I've been grounded by a stroke. I wonder if I'll ever get better.

My right hand doesn't work. I'm forty-six years old, and Mum is feeding me like a baby, one spoonful of soup at a time. Can you imagine how discouraging this feels?

Over the following weeks, reporters discuss plans to re-float the stranded vessel. But the outer shell of her double hull is damaged. The Pasha Bulker is taking on water. Any attempt to move her must occur at high tide, when her buoyancy will require less towing force and lower the risk of her breaking in two. The biggest concern is a fuel leak.

I hope my rehabilitation won't be as fraught. I'm terrified I'll never walk properly again, or regain the use of my right hand. And my speech … what if I never get it back?

But if you think this is going to be a sob story, you're wrong.

This book is about getting painful emotions out of my system so I can move on. It's about my rehabilitation and ongoing recovery. But hopefully, most of all, my story will offer encouragement to other stroke survivors, as well as to anyone else determined to push through adversity and grow stronger.

A MEMOIR OF STROKE, RENEWAL AND THE POWER OF SONG

I WILL

PART 1

LISMORE BASE HOSPITAL

Out of the Blue

It was a Friday that started out like any other. I was feeling a little sick but looking forward to the long weekend. My husband Brad and I were planning to go to Wintersun, a retro nostalgia festival at Coolangatta, which was only an hour north from our home at Alstonvale on the Far North Coast of NSW. Brad's friend Bill Carr would be flying up from Sydney. The three of us were excited about the idea of going to a festival with live music, rock 'n' roll dancing and classic American cars like hot rods and Mustangs.

I was working as a drama teacher at Lismore High School. On the way to school I picked up my friend Linda, who was an art teacher. As Linda hopped into the car she said hello in a very cheery voice. I guessed she was also looking forward to the long weekend. Although I didn't want to dampen Linda's upbeat mood, I told her I wasn't feeling well.

'School's really getting to me,' I said, 'and I'm feeling

exhausted all the time. I'm worried about my marriage and Brad's business. Brad's always right about everything and I'm tired of it. He doesn't want to go to counselling and I'm at my wit's end. I don't know whether to leave or give it another go.'

I also told Linda that my doctor had explained I was anaemic from heavy menstrual bleeding and had sent me to see a gynaecologist. The gynaecologist had prescribed iron injections as well as pills called Cyklokapron and Triphasil, which he said would both help, in their own different ways, to reduce excessive bleeding. At this stage, I didn't think too much about the possible side effects of taking both these drugs simultaneously. I simply did what the doctor ordered.

So, now aged forty-five, I had also agreed to have surgery to have a coil placed in my uterus. The coil would be a hormone-releasing IUD (or Intra-Uterine Device) used not just to prevent pregnancies but also to treat heavy periods. The surgery was scheduled to take place two weeks after the long weekend. 'In the meantime,' the gynaecologist had advised me, 'it's important that you take the pills.'

As we chatted away in the car, Linda was sympathetic. 'Go to Wintersun and relax, but see your doctor when you get back, yeah?'

'Okay,' I agreed. 'I'll get everything sorted after the long weekend.'

We arrived at school. After walking into the main building with Linda, I headed straight to the Drama room, which was across the quadrangle and upstairs in the same building as the English classrooms. I always looked forward to this Friday morning class, as it was my lovely Year Tens. I was relieved that it wasn't my ratty Year Eights; I didn't think I could cope with them while I was feeling so crook.

I opened the classroom door and walked in. One of my favourite students, a dark-haired girl called Hannah, walked in right behind me.

'Hi, Miss. Can I do anything to help you?' she asked.

'No thanks, Hannah,' I said. 'I've got everything covered.'

Then a boy named Oscar arrived.

'Where's that overdue assignment, Oscar?' I asked.

Oscar was intelligent but lazy. I suspected he was doing drama because there weren't too many written assignments.

The boy gave me a disarming smile. 'I left it at home, Miss. But I'll bring it in after the long weekend.'

I was just about to interrogate Oscar when the bell rang.

'Saved by the bell,' I joked. 'Just make sure you get that assignment in by Tuesday or I'll be sending your parents a letter.'

The other students were gathering in the classroom. There were only about twelve of them.

'We'll start with a warm-up,' I said, feeling sicker by the minute. 'Shake your hands, everyone.'

We formed a circle and the kids began shaking their hands.

I was shaking my hands too but something weird began happening. There were spasms in my right hand. I had to stop what I was doing. Then I felt I lost control over my limbs, and even the rest of my body.

It must have looked bad because the students made me sit down. A sea of concerned faces surrounded me. The spasms subsided.

'I'm all right,' I said, trying to make light of the situation.

Some of the students were crying. I heard Hannah say, 'Miss, you're not all right.'

Apparently Oscar ran downstairs to get help, but it seemed like ages before it came. First, there was Judy Tasker, the lady from the office. Judy was the first aid officer, and she assessed my situation. Then she led me down the stairs to the English staff room.

Although I was still insisting I was okay I must have looked very unwell, as my head teacher Dot Huey arrived on the scene. Dot said my Drama students were upset, and that she'd tried to reassure them that I would be fine.

She said she'd told them, 'You can go to the art room. Mrs Myles will take you.' Dot said some poor children didn't want to go, but that they eventually went.

Brad arrived. He said, 'What's all this?'

Despite our differences, I was relieved to see my husband. I held onto his hand.

Judy said, 'Your wife has had a turn and I think we should call an ambulance.'

I looked at Brad expectantly.

'Jenny, how are you feeling?' he asked.

I nodded. 'I'm fine.'

Brad said, 'Well, we'll hop in my car and go the hospital.'

But Dot and Judy weren't happy with that idea. Dot told Brad she was calling an ambulance, and Judy said, 'I think your wife should be checked straight away.'

I was getting worse and now Brad could see that, so he said, 'Okay. I'll follow the ambulance.'

When the ambulance arrived, I was still trying to reassure Brad that I was okay. There were two ambulance officers – a man and a woman – and they began doing all sorts of things and asking me my name. They carried me out of the school on a stretcher. The stretcher, like a bed, even had white sheets. I saw children staring at me. I remember the trip to Lismore Base Hospital. I was confused and worried and frightened. What was happening to me?

The ambulance took me straight to the hospital's Emergency Department. Everyone there was efficient. They gave me a series of tests – I can't remember which ones – but I do recall a doctor shining a light into my eyes and saying, 'What is your name?'

'Jennifer Sheldon,' I said. But that was my old name. I hadn't said my married name: Jennifer Miller. I corrected myself.

I had an angiogram of my head and neck. An angiogram uses x-rays and a special dye to take pictures of blood vessels, and it's good at revealing any blockages or haemorrhages. I also had a CT (or CAT) scan of my brain. The official name for this test is 'computer axial tomography', and it produces cross-sectional images of the body using x-rays and a computer. Both the angiogram and CT scan showed that I had suffered a left CVA, which is short for 'cerebrovascular accident'.

What this means in everyday language is that I had suffered a stroke on the left side of my brain. A stroke is what happens when the blood supply to the brain is interrupted, depriving the brain cells of oxygen. This can happen in two main ways. Either because there is a blood clot that 'obstructs' a blood vessel in the brain (an ischaemic stroke), or due to a blood vessel in the brain that ruptures (an haemorrhagic stroke).

As a specialist called Dr Fiona Wagner later explained to me, I had suffered a minor ischaemic stroke that was caused by an embolus – or blood clot – in my left middle cerebral artery. Dr Wagner said this blood clot had led to some brain tissue damage, which had caused the symptoms I had experienced at school that morning.

But all I vaguely understood at that point was that I had had a minor stroke, and that apparently I was lucky. Doctors said that hospital staff would monitor me overnight.

'No!' I said. I wanted to go home straight away. I argued with everyone about this, but they were adamant that I stay.

Brad rang my parents, who were having morning tea at their home in Sydney, having spent the entire previous day driving all the way down there from their holiday unit in Coolangatta. Mum answered the call and heard Brad say, 'Jenny had a turn.'

Mum said, 'What do you mean? Do you mean she's had a stroke?'

Brad said, 'She's all right. She's reading a magazine.'

Once I was admitted to a ward, Brad came in and spent some time with me. After a while, he kissed me goodbye, promising he would come to take me home the next day. I was pleased at the thought that I would be out of hospital so soon.

A Frightening Night

Then it happened overnight: I had a massive stroke. I almost died. Now I couldn't move on the right side of my body and I couldn't speak.

After an incredibly long night, sunshine began streaming in through a nearby window. I didn't know where I was. I was muddled and frightened.

What was happening to me? I couldn't move my right leg. I couldn't speak. The nurses made me as comfortable as they could, and I waited for Brad.

Eventually, Brad arrived. He was shocked when the doctors told him that I'd had a big stroke during the night – after all, he'd been expecting to take me home.

Of course, I couldn't say anything to him. I tried to. I wanted to reassure him that I was all right but I couldn't. His good friend Bill was coming from Sydney that evening by plane, and I thought that was good because Bill would be a distraction for him.

I was taken for another CT scan. While Brad waited for me to have the scan, he made various calls, mainly to my parents and close friends. My parents were distressed and booked flights for early the next morning, so they could come back up to the Northern Rivers.

Perhaps because the big stroke happened at the beginning of a long weekend, there were no specialists around to examine me. So all I could do after having the second CT scan was wait for my parents to arrive. Fortunately, my head teacher Dot came to visit me that afternoon.

All I was able to say was 'yes', 'no' and 'I don't think so'. I could understand individual words but couldn't follow a whole idea. But Dot was lovely. She didn't freak out. Years earlier, her father had had a stroke, so she had some insight into what I was going on. Dot had brought along some hand cream so she proceeded to put it on my hands. She said everything would be all right, and that a competent teacher would take over my classes. She also told me her mother was praying for me. I had Dot's mother on my side and I liked her a lot. I was really touched.

Then I had another lonely and bewildering night in the hospital. My right leg and arm were frozen. Why couldn't I speak? Why couldn't I move? I was thinking these thoughts but I couldn't speak them.

One Stroke or Two?

The following morning, which was a Sunday, Brad brought Bill in to visit me. Bill was stunned to see what had happened. Another person who came that morning was my dear friend Denise Gerards. Denise and I go way back. Many years ago we had studied together at the Northern Rivers College of Advanced Education. She had also been my bridesmaid. Denise drove down to Lismore from the Gold Coast, and I appreciated that. I was not surprised to see her. She had always been there for me through thick and thin.

Another devoted friend who helped me at that time was Heather Green. I'd met Heather through a local Lions Club and we'd been friends for about a year. Like Bill, Heather looked really shocked when she saw me, but she quickly pulled herself together to offer me emotional and practical support. She fed me tomato soup and was generous of her time with me.

Then Mum and Dad arrived. To say I was relieved to see them would be an understatement.

The doctors told my parents about the results of the second CT scan. Apparently tissue damage could be seen in a part of the brain known as the left basal ganglia. There was also tissue damage in the caudate nucleus, one of the left basal ganglia's main components. As a doctor explained to them: 'Quite a few fibres of nerve cell tracts travel in close proximity through the brain at this area, so a small amount of damage can affect a large part of a person's body.'

Although I don't recall many things from that first weekend in hospital, I do remember a speech therapist coming to see me. She was the one who most clearly explained to me that I had had two strokes: first the little one, then the big one.

Since then, however, I've found that no one in the medical profession can say if I had one stroke or two, mainly because there's so much conjecture about the process and timing of things. As clinical psychologist, author and stroke survivor Dr David Roland would explain to me many years later after looking at the medical notes made by my doctor, 'It's hard to determine whether the effects of the first event were transient as the ensuing event happened soon after, suggesting a causal link.' In other words, he said, 'It's quite possible that the underlying cause of the first event – a blood clot – was the same as for the second event, except that in the second event the effects were major.'

For me, what's tricky in terms of making a choice between referring to a singular 'stroke' or the plural 'two strokes', is that from my perspective I experienced two distinct episodes: a relatively minor one on the Friday morning, and then a big one sometime that night. But for the purposes of my story I'll simply refer to my 'stroke' in the singular. After all, this is what the medicos do.

A Testing Time

Sitting beside my hospital bed, the speech therapist gave me some pictures on cards to help me explain simple things, like when I wanted to go to the toilet. There were also images for emotions, like a sad face for times I was feeling down in the dumps, and an angry face for whenever I was upset. There was also a smiley face. I wondered when on earth I would get to use that.

There were so many tests. I had my swallowing tested, and I could swallow liquids, but that was all. After a few days, I could manage pureed foods.

Bath times were challenging. This was because I was frozen on one side. A nurse took me to a white-tiled bathroom, where she helped me undress before spraying my body with water from a showerhead. She then wiped me down with a cloth. I didn't want to remain like this. I was determined to get better.

A physiotherapist came to see me. She gave me a kind of harness and got me walking around a bit. Mostly, I did a lot of sleeping. Apparently this was part of the recuperative process.

Sooner than I thought, the smiley card came in handy. I had a lot of support. Friends rushed to see me. My Ballina friend Jane Elliot came to visit and she was supportive, telling me that hospital was the best place for me at the moment. And there were visits from cousins and other friends, and flowers from many people I knew, and I was overwhelmed with cards from my students. The nurses told me my students wanted to see me but they had to be content to send the cards. This really touched me. I showed the nurse the smiley card!

But Dad wasn't coping very well. He was getting forgetful in his old age and I was worried about him. He was very upset to see what had happened to me. Bill very kindly took him up to the holiday unit at Coolangatta. I was glad Dad could get a break from the hospital. And one nice thing was that when Dad came back a couple of days later, he presented me with a toy dog. Brad said, 'Let's call her Millie' and that was that. I was so touched that Dad gave me the toy dog that I still have her today. Whenever I feel blue, and whenever I want to feel close to Dad, I hold Millie.

I did use the sad card the most, though. I used it when I felt humiliated after pressing a buzzer in vain. No one came to help me, and I soiled my nappy. I also used the sad card to say how I felt about my shared room. It was noisy in the hospital, and the shared room was stark and bare. There were six beds, so it was hardly private. I had to have the curtain pulled across. A number of medical staff came to see me. I was always being prodded and poked.

There was one woman in my room who called out all the time, even when I was trying to sleep. Eventually, there was an outbreak of something or other, perhaps some kind of gastric thing, and it was contagious but I didn't have it. The nurses shifted me to a private room because I was a private patient.

Bliss! It was so good to have a private room, especially as all I wanted to do was sleep. I had been seriously anaemic again. My gynaecologist performed the minor surgery to insert the IUD, and I was also given a blood transfusion. I felt continually tired.

I remember Brad getting some books for me. They were mainly romance novels and I tried to read them in bed. But I was reading with little comprehension. I could understand words individually but I couldn't follow a whole idea. I couldn't understand what was happening to me. One afternoon, I threw the books across the room – with my left hand, obviously!

A week or so later I did try reading again. This was when Brad's cousins, Matt and Vanessa, drove up from Wollongong to visit me. Vanessa gave me two picture books. I could say every word in the books, but I couldn't put all the words together fluently. Imagine how frustrating that was! I was a school teacher and I couldn't fluently read a children's book. It was devastating. When the speech pathologist asked me about the children's books, I pointed to a card that showed the sad face. I like to think she understood what I was getting at.

Sometimes there were occasions when my emotions were so mixed that I would need to hold up both the sad and smiley faces at the same time. One day when I was in the general ward, for example, I was having a late-afternoon nap when I was woken by loud clanging sounds. A nurse walked into my room and said, 'The Lismore Lantern Parade is here! Do you want to see it?'

I nodded, so the nurse pressed buttons to raise the top

section of my bed, making it easier for me to sit up. This happened just in time for a dragon to appear in my room – a dragon lantern with huge green eyes that seemed to stare right through me! The dragon's body was multi-coloured with red, yellow and white light blazing through it, and inside the dragon were several people. Then came an enormous owl lantern with her wings outspread … and then a huge red heart … and then bright yellow luminous lanterns in the shape of sunflowers. The procession in and out of the room was a whirlwind of chaos. Then suddenly, it was gone.

It was lovely to see a selection of lanterns in the lead-up to the Lismore Lantern Parade, which was set to take place over the following weekend, when it would weave back and forth along the main streets after sunset on the Saturday night. But I also felt sad thinking back to the days when I was part of the parade in the outside world. As a teacher at Lismore High School, I'd often volunteered to help the Year Sevens and some of the older intellectually disabled students to be part of the parade.

I remember some twin boys in particular. They struggled at school but were so happy to be part of the lantern event. I could still see them carrying their red and blue lanterns down the street, running up to me to insist, 'Isn't it awesome, Miss!' with their little faces looking around in wonder. They were so proud of themselves.

Back then I hadn't been aware that a small number of the lantern-bearers always made an effort to visit the hospital. This was a good thing, as so many of the patients needed cheering up. But now, I was one of those patients. I was happy to have seen the lanterns, but also sad that this year I wasn't able to be part of the bigger event outside.

Lovestruck

Now that I had my own room, I could spend a lot more time sleeping. And when I wasn't sleeping, I unfortunately had plenty of time to ponder the problems with my marriage. I believe Brad loved me very much. I loved him, too. And I know this probably sounds crazy, but even though I was stuck in hospital – paralysed on my right side and barely able to speak – I found that I was fretting about Brad more than I was worrying about myself. My husband often looked quite stressed when he came to visit me.

At our wedding just over three years earlier, I'd wanted to believe our life together was going to be a fairy tale. It was April 3, 2004. I got ready at a hotel called Pier One, which is right beside the Sydney Harbour Bridge. The wedding ceremony was held at dusk on a jetty in Balmain – it was the Elliot Street Wharf – and the setting was magical. I travelled there by water taxi, a special one for the wedding. My *Stairwell to Heaven* choir was assembled on the jetty when I arrived, and they sang a few songs, including the Etta James version of *At Last*.

'At last my love has come along,' they sang. 'My lonely days are over, and life is like a song.'

To reach Brad, I walked through an archway covered with green ivy and pink lilies. There were candles everywhere, which is something I had planned. With the fading light, the atmosphere was stunning. We said our vows.

We had our reception in a lovely Greek restaurant, where I'd arranged for a selection of entrées to be served out in the open so I could include the choir in that. Afterwards, we had a sit-down dinner.

I'd first met Brad at Five Dock RSL. I wanted to find someone to have children with. I wanted to meet my soulmate. So in an attempt to do that I went to a ten-week dancing course. As I searched for the man of my dreams, I figured I could learn dancing at the same time. At least if I didn't meet anyone, I wouldn't be wasting my time.

It was on the dance floor that I first saw Brad, and he was small but handsome. He had dark hair and was thickset and he made me laugh. I had a drink with him and he bumped into a friend of his called Narelle, who worked behind the bar there. Narelle sat down to joke with Brad, and it was in that instant that I realised I wanted to get to know him.

It was a whirlwind romance. Brad was living at Drummoyne and I was living at Summer Hill at that time. I was working at Fairfield High School and he had his own printing business. I thought that was awesome and I wanted nothing more than to get to know him. He had grown up in Balmain in a working class family and had managed to have his own business. I was impressed.

Brad was married but had separated from his wife, and now they were getting divorced. He was sad because the split had affected his three teenage children: two girls and one boy. The children hated me, but I decided everything would be okay.

They would resent me at first but life was bound to come good.

In the summer evenings, I liked walking with Brad around Drummoyne, near the water. Many times we would end up at an Italian restaurant that served an excellent banoffee pie, Brad's favourite. Banoffee pie is an English dessert made from bananas, toffee and cream on a pastry base. Yummy!

Our relationship began getting serious. I introduced Brad to my parents. We went touring through the Hunter Valley and also visited Byron Bay. I was falling hard for him. I was smitten. I wanted to marry him.

After about a year and a half, I asked Brad to move in with me. Not long after that, he wound up his printing business and went travelling to the Northern Territory with his best friend Bill. Even though I was in touch with him – I made him call me every night! – I missed him like crazy.

When Brad returned, he began getting depressed over a large sum of money a client owed him. It was becoming a long-term debt. One day, Brad and I went to the client's farm and he said that all he could give Brad was a motorboat. The boat was a far cry from the money, but at least it was something.

We ended up using the motorboat a lot. I encouraged Brad to bring the children out on it. While we were out on the water I told the children how much I wanted to be friends with them but to no avail. The eldest daughter in particular was a 'daddy's girl' and she certainly didn't want to have anything to do with me. I felt very sad for her. I couldn't imagine how it would feel to be sixteen and have your parents getting divorced. My parents were still together after many years and they had a wonderful marriage.

My father was born in Sydney in 1932. His parents named him Bruce Henry Gilbert Sheldon. He studied to be a doctor at the University of Sydney and would go on to become a gynaecologist. My mother was born in Murwillumbah in 1937. She was christened Winsome Gae Godwin, but right from day dot her grandmother started calling her Gae in a pre-emptive strike against anyone calling her Winnie. To my great-grandmother's relief, the name Gae stuck. Everyone calls her Gae!

After Mum qualified as a primary school teacher, she was sent to a small school at Warrilla on the south coat of NSW, and it was there she met my father, when he turned up one day to give needles to the children. Dad fell head over heels in love with Mum at first sight. Mum was engaged to someone else, but she quickly broke it off with that person and married Dad within six months.

Cracks Appear

Some people might assume I became a teacher because I decided to follow in my mother's footsteps. Not true. I had always wanted to be an actor and singer. But during the 1980s, I thought I'd better study teaching so I had something to fall back on whenever I couldn't find enough acting and singing jobs to pay my bills. And here's where life can surprise you: I found that I adored being a teacher!

I studied teaching at the University of New England in Armidale and quickly fell in love with that part of the world. Once I was working in Sydney I often dreamt of going north. After I had married Brad, I thought I would test this idea on him by inviting him up to the Northern Rivers for a holiday with my cousin. Luckily for me that's when he fell in love with the area, too.

Brad and I decided to move there! After signing a six-month lease on a property in Wollongbar, we invited Brad's Uncle Alfie to come and join us. But Uncle Alfie was getting too old and frail. He couldn't come.

Uncle Alfie was such an important person in our lives. He had raised Brad – mainly because his sister was Brad's mother, and she had been an alcoholic. Uncle Alfie was a lovely man; he was very kind and considerate. I became very fond of him. Once, when Brad and I had just returned from our honeymoon in Fiji, my brother John and his wife Kirsty had their first baby, Jack. Uncle Alfie was sick in hospital at the time and really wanted to see the baby. I thought it was lovely that the baby was so important to him.

Sadly, Uncle Alfie never got to see Jack. He became even sicker. Brad and I ended up taking home his small dog, a Cavalier King Charles Spaniel by the name of Splat – such a beautiful dog. Then Uncle Alfie died and that was when some very stressful times began.

Uncle Alfie had three sisters, including Brad's mother, and Brad began arguing with them – over the will, and over the funeral arrangements … over everything, really. I didn't much admire the way Brad was constantly arguing with his aunts, but he was upset at losing Alfie, so I just told myself it was the grief speaking.

Then things got worse. Uncle Alfie had left his house to Brad and Brad's cousin Matt. The two of them wanted to sell the house but one of the aunts was living in it and she wouldn't budge. The aunts ended up taking us to court. Even though we eventually settled the conflict through mediation, the entire process was horrible and Brad really wasn't coping.

One day, I was at a friend's place for a special dinner. Brad was there, too. He became really drunk and started getting aggressive with another guest, who happened to be one of my former bosses. I got Brad out of the house as quickly as I could, but as we were driving away he became even more aggressive, wanting to fight someone. At an intersection, when a window washer approached us, Brad nearly got out of the car. He wanted to fight the window washer!

I should have been warned by all this aggression, but I genuinely thought it was a result of all the build-up of stress Brad had experienced from getting divorced, trying to get clients to pay debts, dealing with Uncle Alfie's death, and battling with his aunts over his inheritance.

Once the inheritance money came through, we bought a farm with it. The farm was at Alstonvale, which is very close to Wollongbar, where we'd been renting. We had a mortgage, but we felt the farm was going to set us up for the rest of our lives. Brad actually decided we were going to go into worm farming, and that as a sideline he would also sell eco-friendly composting systems that used fermented organic matter to eliminate odours while the food was decomposing. It was a good idea.

Meanwhile, I found my dream job teaching Drama and English at Lismore High School. But even though it was my dream job, the work was very demanding. Also, outside of teaching, I helped Brad with his business. We went to markets to sell the worms and composting systems. I was fairly good at selling them. Even though I didn't get much rest, I was happy Brad's business was going well.

School was stressful. Home was stressful. As soon as I got home from school I would have to do things around the house. I thought that was all just part of marriage. Also, at various times two of Brad's children also came to live with us. This never worked out.

One time when Brad's son was living with us over some summer holidays, Mum and Dad had driven north to stay with us as well. Brad was cooking spaghetti bolognaise and he wanted some basil. We didn't have any, and Brad lost his temper. He called me all sorts of names and broke our kitchen rubbish bin. My parents were worried about me but I reassured them everything would be all right.

Once my parents had left, I looked around the community for something Brad could take an interest in. He was in the house a lot. I finally hit on Lismore SES. This was successful at first because it got Brad out of the house. I would go along with him. One day, though, I didn't go. It was the first day after the SES had given us some uniforms that were much too large. Brad had a go at the person in charge and that was the end of our time there.

Brad was like Jekyll and Hyde. He could be very loving to me one minute and then turn on me the next. He was a very angry man. I sometimes thought this was because he had abandonment issues with his mother, and I felt determined to make our marriage work. If I showed him enough love, everything would be all right.

But I was always walking on eggshells. I kept changing my behaviour to suit him. There were so many upsetting incidents that it would take me an entire book to describe them all, but one that sticks in my mind was when Brad and I were staying at my parents' place in Sydney. Dad was dying. He had cancer. So it was already a stressful time without Brad adding to it.

I was making a curry, and Brad decided to help me. He was agitated. I had seen this kind of agitation simmering away before, so I was wary and tried to jolly him along. Mum and Dad were downstairs in the rumpus room and I was alone in the kitchen with Brad. There were some vegetables out on the chopping board and I was trying to cut an onion. I could feel Brad watching me and I was nervous. There had been so many times he had admonished me for cutting onions the wrong way. It always caused him grief; I don't know why.

Anyway, I cut the onion. Brad was so angry that he punched me in the arm. I was shocked. I didn't know what to say. I bruise easily and it left a bruise. I was afraid that Mum and Dad would notice later, but they didn't say anything. They were too worried about Dad's health. Dad had been so sick with various ailments, and now he also had bowel cancer, which was what had killed by brother Mark. So my dear parents were still grieving that huge loss while also dealing with Dad's declining health. Naturally, I wanted to protect them from the problems I was having with Brad.

So Many Challenges

In 2007, some days after my stroke, a lovely nurse called Jean told me that even though I would be leaving the hospital in a couple of days, I wouldn't be going home. Instead, I was going to be transferred to a state-of-the-art rehabilitation service in the nearby coastal town of Ballina.

I had come to depend on Jean. On the night I was moved to my own room, I had been feeling really depressed and at one stage was close to tears. Jean was just coming into my room with my dinner on a tray. Noticing the expression on my face, she had started to make a fuss of me.

'Jenny, anything you want you just press this buzzer and I will come running,' is what she had said.

Then she went about cheering me up. She definitely knew how to make me feel good.

Anyway, it was Jean who helped me get my head around the idea of going to rehab. She talked to my family about how we could borrow a wheelchair from the hospital, so they could take me over to Lismore Shopping Square for what we thought of as a 'buying expedition' to prepare for Ballina Rehab. I wanted to get a tracksuit and some slippers, as well as a few other things.

My parents decided we would go across the road to the square on my final Sunday in hospital, as that was the day before I would go to Ballina, and it was also when the car boot markets would be on. So on that Sunday morning Mum, Dad, Brad and my friend Denise wheeled me across the road and down the street to do some shopping. For a couple of years,

Brad and I had operated a market stand to sell his composting systems and worm farms, so I knew a lot of other stall holders there. I remember the shock on their faces when they saw me, as they hadn't even heard that I had had a stroke.

That night, all I could think about was going to rehab the next morning. I didn't know what to expect. For a while, I tried to take my mind off things by watching television, but that didn't work. I decided I would press the buzzer for my favourite nurse Jean, to see if she could help me go to the toilet now so I wouldn't need to call anyone in the middle of the night. Jean came straight away and helped me to the bathroom. Afterwards, she settled me back into bed and said, 'Now, you get a good night's sleep.'

But I couldn't sleep. I tossed and turned. I started feeling frightened. I wanted my parents or my husband. *Stop this*, I told myself silently. *You are going to Ballina Rehab and you are going to get better.* But then I started to cry, and suddenly Jean was there. She held my hand. I was so grateful. She was an angel and watched over me throughout the night.

PART 2

BALLINA REHAB

Personal Care

I had to get better! Late in the afternoon on Monday June 18, a wardsman from Lismore drove me to Ballina District Hospital, where a state-of-the-art rehabilitation unit had just opened. The moment I was wheeled into my own room, I let out a sigh of relief. Everything was brand new. The room had an ensuite and sitting room. It was peaceful.

But within half an hour, my good mood disappeared. Two nurses moved me from my wheelchair into a regency chair – a large mobile chair that reclines, and that you can stay sitting in for long periods. I knew these chairs were only for people with high care needs. I felt awful.

Brad and my parents arrived. They all admired the chair, impressed that I could remain sitting in it quite comfortably once someone had wheeled me to another place. Dad demonstrated by pushing me into the dining room for dinner.

This was when I saw the Pasha Bulker on the TV and

realised ten days had passed since my stroke. Mum fed me my dinner, and afterwards Brad wheeled me back to my room. The whole time, I stayed in my chair.

My husband and parents said goodbye, and a nurse got me ready for bed. I was exhausted. I slept the sleep of the dead.

Rehab was hard. I was depressed at first. The nurses did everything for me, including giving me a bath – and this really grated on me. One nurse singled me out for attention. With her bouncy blonde ponytail and a personality to match, she was very friendly. Too friendly.

'Hi, I'm Gail, and I'm going to be your personal nurse!' she beamed at me the first time we met.

I couldn't speak so I simply smiled at her.

'Let's get you in the shower!' was her next comment.

Gail found a shower chair and bustled me into it. She removed the sling from my right arm and got me out of my clothes. After turning on the shower and taking great pains to make sure the water temperature was just right – chatting non-stop as she fiddled with the settings – she used the hand-held shower nozzle to give me a very thorough wash.

Gail then dried me with a white hospital towel. 'We'll have to get some talcum powder for you. Will Lily of the Valley be all right?'

I nodded.

She then helped me into my underpants and bra. How I wished I could still do those simple things for myself. Now I was sitting self-consciously on the bed dressed in nothing more than my underwear.

Gail flicked through the garments hanging sadly in the wardrobe. 'Let's see, how about we put you into a tracksuit? I believe you're off to the gym! So yes, it will have to be a tracksuit. We have a couple of tracksuits here, so why don't you pick the colour?'

By now I was out of my wheelchair and able to walk slowly and tentatively. Gail was holding up my pink tracksuit, so again I nodded.

Once I'd been 'popped into' my exercise gear, I took hold of the arm Gail held out to me and allowed her to escort me to the dining room. 'Ooh, I wonder what's for morning tea?' she rattled on.

I was in despair. Imagine not being able to shower!

From that day, Gail showered me every morning. Gradually, I could feel myself getting physically stronger. I longed for the moment I could have a shower on my own.

Gail was very kind to me, so I tried to be patient, but suddenly one morning I had had enough. Once Gail had me out of the shower and dressed, she began brushing my hair. As usual, she was talking non-stop. Perhaps I was feeling pretty down in the dumps that day, because before I could stop myself I raised my left arm and grabbed the hairbrush from her hand.

'No!' I said angrily, attempting to brush my hair myself.

A minute later, when I had given up, Gail said quietly, 'You look lovely, Jenny. I'll help you to the gym.'

But I was feeling overly emotional and stormed from the room as quickly as I could, which meant that I was probably moving pretty slowly. I lurched down the corridor – straight past the gym and all the way through the automatic glass doors and out into the cold winter air. Boy, did I feel sorry for myself. I was cross with Gail but couldn't express this adequately. I knew she had my best interests at heart, and that she was a caring and decent person. But I was just so fed up with all the chattering, and I was sick and tired of needing help with my personal care requirements.

After a few minutes out in the cold, I shuffled back to my room and sat on my bed.

Gail looked in on me. 'Are you okay?'

I nodded.

'Well,' she said in a very subdued voice, 'as long as you are.' And then she walked away.

Out and About

While at Ballina Rehab, my support team encouraged me to go on short outings with friends and family. On the first Saturday I was there, Brad came to take me on a lunch date. Even though I had no idea where we were going, I was excited. I was glad to be going out with Brad.

The venue turned out to be the Ballina RSL. I was happy just to be out of rehab – even if only for a couple of hours. Brad helped me out of his truck and we carefully made our way across the carpark and passed through the club's automatic glass doors. They opened like magic. I was feeling good! But then a staff member asked me to sign into the club. Confusion! There was no way I could sign the register with my right hand. My right hand was paralysed from the stroke. It was in a sling. Turning to Brad, I was suddenly teary.

'You can do it with your left hand,' he suggested, before explaining to the staff member that I had suffered a stroke.

So I signed in with my left hand. My writing felt wonky, and my signature looked like a little scribble.

I then proceeded up the stairs, holding onto Brad for dear life. Getting to our table took a massive effort. Once we were seated, I told Brad I would love to order a pasta dish. I wanted to be normal. I could eat pasta. Brad went to a counter to order and it seemed like forever before he was back. He handed me some wine but I couldn't drink it. I had always enjoyed wine, but now it tasted strange. This confused me.

At this point, one of Brad's friends was walking by and noticed us. He said he was sorry to hear I'd had a stroke. Brad began to tell him my entire story. This seemed to go on for ages. I wanted to sleep. Then when the man finally left, Brad said he would take me back to our place for a visit. He was being nice to me, so I couldn't bring myself to tell him how exhausted I was, and that all I wanted to do was go to bed. I went along with his plans.

Brad got me back into the truck with great difficulty. He then said he'd better check with rehab about taking me to our house and as we drove to Ballina Rehab on the way, I dozed off. When we arrived he told me, 'You can't see the house. I'm so sorry. They need to do an assessment on the house first.'

Relief! I was secretly pleased but pretended to be disappointed. He got me out of the car with great difficulty, and led me back to my room. I needed to sleep. I slept!

Physiotherapy

Learning to walk was hard. I started therapy on my first full day in rehab, which was a Monday. Someone said my physiotherapist would be a woman named Lisa. But Lisa had Mondays off. So I began my rehab with someone else. This was how I met Carmen.

When Carmen first saw me, I was struggling to walk with a cane. She asked if she could give me a hand. All I could say was, 'No. Yes.' Talking was just as hard as walking.

Fortunately Carmen decided 'yes' was my answer! She fetched another walking stick and demonstrated the best way to use it. I tried to copy her and failed. She made me try again.

'This time, put more weight on your right side,' she said.

I began to topple over. Carmen kept me upright. This gave me confidence.

Even though most people I've met since my stroke wouldn't know it, I have a wide vocabulary. As I followed Carmen's instructions, my head filled with uplifting words and phrases: *single-minded; tenacious; resilient; resolute; determined.* Although I couldn't say these words out loud, there was nothing to stop me turning them over in my mind. I suddenly felt excited about the possibility of one day being able to walk as normally as before.

Carmen kept on with her encouragement. 'That's right, more to the left.'

I got better at walking with the cane.

'This time, put more weight on your right side.'

I continued to practice. By the end of that session, I was

able to walk slowly with the cane. I was walking! What a relief.

After my session with Carmen it was time for lunch, but I could barely keep my eyes open. Learning to use the cane had drained me of energy. I desperately needed to sleep, so I skipped lunch and went back to bed. A few hours later, Brad and my parents arrived, and I was able to demonstrate my new skill. They were very impressed. I walked around with them in the corridors of the rehab unit. But before long it was the same old story: I was getting tired, so they fed me and left.

The next morning, I got to meet Lisa, who would be my regular physiotherapist, and Rose, my speech therapist. Lisa was short and slim with red hair and freckles. Rose was a brunette. She was slender and tall. As they made small talk, Lisa and Rose helped me into a wheelchair and took me to an exercise room.

Lisa, as I would eventually discover, was a good physiotherapist. But that day, as she put me through my paces, we had a very difficult session. I couldn't communicate, and felt exasperated. I was lying on the floor. Lisa gave me instructions and I understood them, but my body was writhing all over the place. It wouldn't obey the commands. Our time together sounded a bit like this.

Lisa: Sit up, Jenny.

Me: Ahh.

Lisa: Sit up.

Me: Ahh. Ahh …

When Lisa asked me to move to the right, I couldn't do it, and I couldn't tell her that I couldn't do it. Meanwhile, Lisa and Rose talked over the top of me like I didn't exist. Did they think I was stupid? Perhaps these two had already given up on me? This thought made me angry, but also determined. Not only was I going to walk; I would also get my speech back.

Weightless and Buoyant

I did physiotherapy every day. It was hard. My life seemed to be all about lying on the floor doing stretches, and using a set of parallel bars so I could safely practice my walking. I also did balancing exercises, as well as strength-building exercises for my legs and arms. I could tolerate these tasks, but there was one I really hated: doing star jumps while Lisa made me count out loud. I didn't like that at all. The counting part confused me. I would get the 'one, two, three, four, five' right, and then I would forget, and I would have to start again from the beginning. It maddened me that I couldn't get to ten.

So no, my favourite type of physiotherapy was definitely not star jumps. My favourite physiotherapy was swimming! I remember going swimming at lot at a nearby aged care facility where there was a heated pool. The day Lisa first told me we were going there I was so excited!

As a child I had suffered from bronchitis, an inflammation of the lungs that caused me to have a horrible cough. I was only about two and a half years old when the coughing began. I remember going to see the doctor and having to get up on the examination table. The doctor would hold up a candle and it was my job to blow it out; then I would get a lollypop. Back home, Mum would lie me down on my stomach over a divan and pat my back quite hard, over and over, in an effort to clear my lungs.

Dad thought swimming would help, so he took me to a pool on the South Coast of NSW, where I learnt to dog paddle, tread water and float on my back. I loved it. Then when my family moved to Sydney in the late-1960s, Dad introduced me to the Olympic pool in the pretty riverside suburb of Carss Park. On most trips there, he brought my brother Mark along as well, but my favourite times were when Dad took me by myself. One day I was swimming around when some boys threw a large rock into the pool. I remember Dad getting me out of the water and telling the boys off.

But while my lungs did become stronger, the cold winters in Sydney weren't helping my cough. Dad was a general practitioner but when he wanted to study obstetrics, he and Mum decided we would all move to Darwin which had a better climate for my bronchitis. It was a good decision. I was seven at the time, and the warmer climate helped me make a complete recovery.

In Darwin, Mark and I got into competitive swimming at the Nightcliff Pool. What a beautiful place to swim! I learnt to do a mean freestyle there. The pool is right on the Nightcliff Foreshore and overlooks Darwin Harbour. Swimming at Nightcliff Pool made me feel like I was on an island holiday … minus the saltwater crocodiles and deadly box jellyfish that live in the nearby ocean!

I was eleven when our family moved back to Sydney, and how lucky for me that Mum and Dad bought a house right near the pool at Carss Park, my favourite place to swim. For most of its history, which I think has covered at least the past fifty or more years, the pool has been known as 'the Olympic Pool Carss Park'. But most people just called it the Carss Park pool, and now Mark and I could walk there if we felt like it.

I loved this pool! Close to bushland and overlooking the Georges River, it was a 1950s-style venue. You walked through a grand entrance to reach the main Olympic pool, and there were rows and rows of seating all around it. There was also a baby pool, and palm trees and lovely lush lawns. And there were kookaburras and loud screeching sulphur-crested cockatoos everywhere, as well as welcome swallows dipping into the water, and rainbow lorikeets streaking by in bright flashes of orange, blue and green.

And who was Dick Caine, you may ask? Well, he trained seventeen world champions in swimming and other sporting events. These champions included the swimmer Michelle Ford (who won gold and bronze medals at the 1980 Moscow Olympics), the marathon swimmer Susie Maroney, the ironman Chris McCormack, as well as boxers Kostya Szyu, Jeff Fenech and Anthony Mundine, and even the St George Dragons rugby league team.

Dick also taught local children how to swim, and throughout his long career at the pool even found time to clean the toilets and mow the grass. I knew he was telling the truth when he said to a local newspaper reporter in 2015, 'Forget the champions, it's the thousands of kids I have coached who have made it so special. I love the kids and I hope they think I am more than just a coach. We are like a family.'

I remember Dick as a short and stocky guy who was an excellent coach. When I got to the pool after school I would jump straight into the cold water and start doing freestyle, and boy did I train! One day Dick was teaching me to do tumble turns, which are used when competitive swimmers reach the end of the swimming pool but still have more lengths to swim. Dick watched me do a tumble turn and said, 'Good work, Jenny!' He then pointed to another swimmer. 'Can you please now teach Jessie? She hasn't gotten the hang of it yet.'

I was filled with pride. Dick thought I was good enough to train other kids!

Funny what you remember. When I was swimming at the Carss Park pool, I always felt I was at one with the water – buoyant and calm. I could get rid of my stress, get it all out. If I'd just had a bad day at school, I couldn't wait to get into the water. This feeling hasn't changed as I've grown up. After a long day, I'll go swimming to keep fit and also to keep calm! Swimming still has the same effect on me; it relaxes me, and makes me happy.

So my family and friends weren't surprised to hear that after my stroke, I so much wanted to go swimming. The first time Lisa took me to the pool for physiotherapy – hydrotherapy! – I couldn't stop smiling. A carer had also come along to the pool, and she helped me change into my swimming costume. As soon as I was changed, I headed straight for the water, preparing to jump in, just as I always had when training at Carss Park. But the carer stopped me.

'No, Jenny,' she said. 'You're no allowed to get in without Lisa.'

I thought the carer was being overly cautious; the pool didn't look very deep. But I shrugged it off in an effort to be polite. So be it. While I waited for Lisa to get changed, I watched several people who were already in the pool doing their exercises. They were all senior citizens. They were laughing and splashing. I wanted to join them.

Finally, Lisa jumped in. I followed a second later. Instantly, I felt weightless and buoyant! I remembered the freedom. It was blissful. Then Lisa put me through some exercises. I recollect it was difficult but I was excited about returning to swimming. I wanted to get back to doing freestyle!

Every time we went to the pool, my swimming improved. I felt like I was getting somewhere. It helped that Lisa made me feel normal. After only a few sessions at the pool, Lisa and I started going by ourselves, without the carer. One morning, when we went into the change room together, Lisa asked me if I was right to change into my swimming costume by myself.

'Yes!' I said. I was determined to do it myself. And I found I was able to.

Aphasia

Rehab was where I learnt about aphasia. Apparently I had it. My speech therapist, Rose, explained that aphasia is a language difficulty caused by damage to the brain. If you have aphasia, you basically have difficulty talking and understanding what other people say, as well as problems with reading, writing, using numbers, and making gestures.

As Rose explained, 'People with aphasia often know what they want to say, but have trouble getting their messages out.' Wow. Despite Rose's habit of talking to other health professionals in my presence as though I wasn't there, it seemed that she did, after all, have some idea of the frustration I was experiencing.

It was validating to have a name for my problem. Aphasia. I knew what I wanted to say but had trouble getting it out! Thank goodness I could now read – at least I wouldn't have to learn how to do that again. I had enough to re-learn. After three weeks in rehab I could walk without the cane and after two weeks I could deliver several more words than when I first arrived. At that point, all I'd been able to say were three basic statements: 'Yes', 'No' and 'I don't think so'.

But more than anything else, what I was learning in rehab was how to be patient. I began thinking of myself as a patient patient! I enjoyed the pun. At least I hadn't lost my sense of humour.

The Word 'Rabbit'

Rose and I began getting along well. We now seemed to be on the same page. With my spirits buoyed, I was resolute. I was going to get my speech back! I wanted to be able to have proper conversations. Rose was the right person to help me, so I did everything she said. We had a routine; Rose would come to get me from the dining room after breakfast, and sometimes after lunch as well.

For our sessions, she would take me to a special room designed for speech therapy. There was a giant clock on the wall, and I attempted to tell the time. I found this exercise frustrating as I understood what the clock was telling me but couldn't find a way to express the information.

Rose also gave me exercises with flash cards. On each card was a picture of an everyday object or subject, such as a fork, knife, spoon, girl or boy. One by one, Rose would take out the cards and patiently ask, 'What's this?'

I'd see a rabbit, for example, and know exactly what it was. But I couldn't say the word.

Rose would prompt me. 'R ... Rab ...'

And eventually I would get it. 'Rabbit!'

Being able to say a word like 'rabbit' gave me a great sense of achievement. Responding to the flash cards was hard work, but I was making progress.

The result of this progress was that Rose began to bring out more difficult flash cards: ones that required me to describe positions, such as left, right, over, under, down and on top. I was surprised to find how difficult I found these new cards, which required me to say phrases, like 'cage over canary'. I became frustrated. I could say a noun like 'canary', for example, but not a preposition such as 'over'. It took me a long time to succeed at this task.

Several years later, Rose would tell me about her perceptions of my time at Ballina Rehab, saying that when she first met me, I presented as teary and frustrated.

'You were impulsive as a result of your stroke,' she said, 'and that was impacting on your communication and actions. I would've described your speech as halting, and you largely spoke in single words. You could say your name – but gave your maiden name – and your occupation. You could repeat words but could not initiate much on your own.'

Rose would remember that when I first came to rehab, I was able to understand simple yes/no questions but had great difficulty saying yes or no. 'Often you would say both. This caused you frustration but you continued to try until you got it right. Every time! You never gave up.'

Apparently I was able to follow simple commands such as, 'Touch your nose!', but not longer ones like, 'Touch your nose and shut your eyes!' She said that often I would just repeat the first part of the command.

Rose would also remind me what my writing and reading skills were like. 'You were attempting to write some words with your left hand. You could write some letters in your name but perseverated on these, meaning you wrote the same letters repetitively. When reading, you were able to understand single words but had difficulty comprehending sentence-level written information. You read lots of books on the ward as part of your therapy.'

False Hope?

As I was working with Rose every day, I had to admit I adored her. I learnt to trust her approach to my recovery, and had come to respect her work ethic and honesty.

One afternoon a couple of weeks into my course of intensive speech therapy, Brad and I were chatting with Rose in the corridor outside my room. I announced I couldn't wait to teach again.

Rose looked concerned. 'Jenny, I think that returning to

your career might be unrealistic.'

I replied quite firmly, 'But I *am* going to teach again.'

I thought I was doing fairly well with my rehabilitation, and felt optimistic about one day returning to my old job.

Rose looked at me kindly. 'Jenny, you very well may teach again one day, but it would be unrealistic of me to give you false hope.'

I listened in shock as she continued. 'You know what you want to say, but you can't get it out. Remember, you have aphasia. You could get a lot better, but I honestly don't think you'll return to full-time teaching.'

I felt devastated. My hopes crumbled as Rose kept talking, perhaps in an effort to soften the blow. 'Don't get me wrong, you're making great strides, Jenny – but you have a long way to go. You can't magically dive back into your career overnight. Just keep up the good work and take pride in how well you're doing.'

Rose said goodbye to Brad, squeezed my arm as a parting gesture, and then turned and walked away. As I watched her disappear around the corner, I made a silent promise to myself. I was going to teach again. I would not let anything stop me.

Ups and Downs

I first met my physiotherapist, Narelle, when she came into my room at seven o'clock one morning. While introducing herself and asking me how I was doing, she casually picked up the packet of Weet-Bix from my breakfast tray, opened it for me and breezily tossed the cereal into my bowl.

I studied this new person in my life. She was blonde, small and dynamic. I liked her immediately and nodded to indicate that yes, I was doing well.

'Excellent,' Narelle said. 'Well, we have some tests to do today, so once you've had your shower I'll come and get you.' Then off she went.

That was the day the first of many tests began. One test involved drawing a house. Apparently I tried to draw a house with a chimney and a path – and this drawing was all over the place. But the thing is, I don't remember ever doing that drawing. It's something I would find out about later. What I do recall about those early days with Narelle was that she gave me puzzles to do, and I enjoyed those.

Narelle also showed me how to do tracing exercises in a little booklet. On each page of the booklet were letters of the alphabet.

Narelle said, 'See? On the left-hand page you trace over letters, and then on the adjacent page you try writing the letters on your own.'

I tried tracing a letter using my right hand. It was difficult to do. I felt like a child learning to write for the first time. *But this is therapeutic*, I told myself. *Keep practicing and you'll get somewhere.*

I worked with Narelle nearly every day. I felt that she knew I was intelligent, and that she empathised with my frustration. She always had my best interests at heart. On the days when I was feeling really low she would go the extra mile to cheer me up, often by taking me out to the nearby Cherry Street Café for coffee.

Before long, I realised Narelle had a knack for finding ways to take advantage of these outings by including some occupational therapy. She would ask me to order the coffee. This was a surprisingly hard thing for me to do. It went like this.

Narelle: Ask for a coffee, Jenny. Ask for a flat white.

Me: Coffee.

Waitress: Which one? You can order a flat white, a cappuccino, and a latte …

Me: A flat white.

Waitress: What size would you like? There's small, regular and large.

Me: Large.

I went through this process many times until I finally got it – although I still find ordering coffee a difficult thing to do!

Once I could order coffee without too much trouble, Narelle switched our focus to personal care routines. Aware that I was significantly impaired on the right side of my body, she lectured me on the importance of re-training not only my right arm, but also my way of seeing, so that I could begin to perform many of the basic tasks I once took for granted. I remember looking only at the left side of my body, for instance, but never looking right.

'Practice scanning from left to right, Jenny,' Narelle said. 'Look at your right side when you pull on your pants.'

It was hard to believe, but since having the stroke I had been ignoring the entire right side of my body!

Later, towards the end of my time in rehab, Narelle asked me to once again draw a house. This second time around, I drew a pretty little house with its path and chimney in exactly the right places – and that's when Narelle showed me my original drawing, the one I had no recollection of doing.

The drawing was a mess! The chimney wasn't even connected to the house, but seemed to be floating off towards the far left side of the page like a lonely box-shaped cloud.

I was shocked at the difference between the two drawings, but also relieved that at least my drawings were now making sense, and that I was now aware of what I was doing.

But not every aspect of my thinking was improving. Around that time, some tradesmen were fixing an air-conditioner in the rehab room, and they were making a lot of noise. Terrible! Narelle said I would need to get used to loud noise, but I found this very difficult.

When I couldn't stand the noise for a moment longer, I escaped into my room and shut the door behind me. But I could still hear the workmen, who seemed to be making even more of a racket. As I lay on my bed fighting back tears, I thought back to my days in the classroom, remembering how noisy everyone was – especially in Drama classes, with all the students constantly chattering and yelling. Perhaps Narelle was right, after all. Maybe the thought of going back to teaching was an unrealistic dream.

Making Friends

I tried not to worry too much about the future, and it helped that my days were busy. My schedule went something like this: breakfast at seven and a shower at eight before heading over to the gym for physiotherapy and occupational therapy; lunch at midday; and speech therapy in the afternoon.

During my free time in the early evening, I was withdrawn at first and wanted to stay in my room as much as possible, but the director of nursing coaxed me into socialising. Gradually, I came out of my shell.

My first friend in rehab was a kind old man. Our friendship began early one night when he said hello to me in the dining room. He was talkative and didn't seem to mind my long silences. I noticed that he sought me out night after night, and his willingness to keep me company helped me regain a little more confidence around people.

I became open to the idea of making friends with someone else: a young man who had been beaten up in Lismore. The two of us began playing chess, and even though the young man was suffering from a traumatic brain injury as a result of the attack, he won every game. I didn't mind. Playing chess gave me practice at thinking and visualising, as I continually needed to figure out how I would move my pieces on the board.

When we first started playing, I was often unable to move the chess pieces in ways that matched my intentions. The discrepancy between how I visualised my moves and the moves I actually made was a real eye-opener! I have always had a competitive spirit, so would concentrate intently. Seeing a chance to strategically move my bishop, for example, I would imagine moving the piece in a diagonal direction across the light-coloured squares. But when it came to physically making the move, my hand would cross over onto the dark-coloured squares, sometimes even moving in a horizontal or vertical direction.

'You can't do that,' my opponent would gently explain. 'The bishop moves diagonally, and you're meant to stay within the light brown squares.' He would then patiently demonstrate this move two or three times, to make sure I understood.

But I did understand. The bishop is a powerful piece in chess, and I knew I was supposed to move it only along diagonal lines. What I didn't understand was the disrupted line of communication between my body and brain. What was happening to me? This conundrum became a guiding question for me on my road to recovery. I continued to play chess with my easy-going new friend, and felt happy when my perseverance paid off and the moves I made mirrored my intentions.

A less demanding pastime during my time in rehab was watching *The Bold and the Beautiful* on TV every weekday afternoon. I got hooked on the melodramatic soap opera about the lives of wealthy families in Los Angeles, the stories of their love affairs, scandals and betrayals.

The reason I started watching the show was because I was intrigued by Edith, an elderly resident in our centre who had purple hair, which she wore in a tall bouffant style. At first, I didn't like Edith. She was bossy and argumentative, especially when it came to who watched what on TV.

At around four every afternoon, another resident, Elsie, would say she wanted to watch *Sale of the Century*, but Edith wouldn't budge from her routine.

'No. We have to watch the *The Bold and the Beautiful*,' she'd say. 'Ridge is about to discover his secret daughter.'

I'd sit quietly, trying to mind my own business. I'd feel sorry for Elsie, who was lovely and treated me like her granddaughter – but secretly, I'd be pleased that she wasn't going to be allowed to change the channel.

Elsie would then mutter under her breath, 'Why does bloody Edith get to decide what everyone watches?'

But over time, my view of Edith softened. I could see she was unhappy and didn't have control over her health. I figured that was why she tried to throw her weight around when it came to the television. Edith had moved from a lovely big house to a small room in the rehab centre. I could see how much trouble she was having adjusting, and, deep down, I think she knew she would never again be going home.

Edith must have sensed that I empathised with her, and that I liked her. She started being nice to me, and was protective of me. When it was time for her to move straight from rehab into an aged care centre, I was sad to see her go. Edith had an interesting way about her; she was fierce on the outside and soft on the inside. We had a send-off party for her in the dining room, and I gave her a kiss goodbye.

I also remember an elderly Chinese woman, Yu Yan, who was proud that her son was a doctor. Yu Yan always seemed very worried about me, perhaps because I couldn't talk. And talking, I soon learnt, was one of her favourite activities. Sometimes she told me interesting things, such as details about the history of her name. Apparently 'Yu Yan' was drawn from the phrase 'Yu Xiao Yan Ran', which describes women who have beautiful smiles. I liked that. But mostly, my new acquaintance simply talked and talked and talked without seeming to say very much. I envied Yu Yan her ability to communicate her thoughts with such attention to detail.

Yu Yan was small and slight, and was always asking rapid-fire questions. She reminded me of a little sparrow continually on the search for crumbs of gossip and knowledge. But even though her constant chatter made me tired, she inspired me. She was in rehab after a fall – and like me, she had to learn to walk again. Every day, for an hour at a time, I saw her slowly putting one foot in front of the other on the footpath outside the main building. Her commitment inspired me, reminding me to practice my own physiotherapy exercises.

One day Yu Yan and I were in the rehabilitation room together. She was testing herself on a set of corner training stairs – up and down, up and down. I was doing some very slow walking between two bright orange plastic traffic cones – back and forward, back and forward. As I still couldn't walk well, I was feeling highly determined to make this exercise count. I'd managed to walk back and forward three times when I sensed someone watching me. It was Yu Yan.

'You're getting the hang of it!' she said, clapping her hands in delight.

I looked up at her and smiled, which was all the encouragement she needed to inform me, 'I am ninety!'

Yu Yan was now looking at me expectantly, probably waiting for me to show my astonishment and say she looked much younger. All I could manage, though, was a simple and very low key, 'No.'

'Yes! I am doing really well!' she exclaimed.

As I attempted another lap between the traffic cones, I could hear Yu Yan's voice in the background, seeking approval and attention. She had quickly changed the topic.

'My son is doing very well, also. My son, who is doctor! Not easy to raise son to be doctor. I scrape and save for him. Scrape and save.'

I had taken only four awkward steps when the subject changed again, just as quickly as before. 'What matter with you?'

As I still couldn't say anything more than 'yes', 'no' and 'I don't think so', I could offer Yu Yan no answer.

My silence only made her more insistent. After repeating her original question several times, she slightly rephrased it. 'What wrong with you?'

I wanted to focus on my walking, but Yu Yan was a big distraction. I was on the verge of tears when Narelle, my occupational therapist, came to my rescue. I had been concentrating so hard on my exercises that I had forgotten she was in the room.

'Okay, you guys,' Narelle suddenly said. 'There's too much talking going on.'

I looked over at her and she gave me an apologetic smile.

'Come on, Jenny,' she said. 'I have something else for you to do.'

As Narelle took me by the arm and gently guided me from the room, my heart flooded with gratitude for her empathy and understanding. Seeing that I was teetering on the edge of an emotional meltdown, she had kindly come to my rescue.

At the time I was in rehab, the facility was also home to several men with Type 1 Diabetes. Some had had their legs amputated. These guys were doing it tough and working hard to be normal. But they weren't what most people would consider normal. I recall one man who had a long straggly beard and a tall lanky body to match. His name was Steve and he slept in the room opposite mine. One of his legs had been cut off at the knee.

I remember having a conversation with Steve in his room. I had wandered in there to say hello but he was the one who spoke first.

'How are you going?' he asked.

I nodded. 'Hi,' was all I managed to say.

But Steve was kind. 'That's the way!' he replied in an encouraging tone.

He noticed I was looking at a portrait of his wife and children.

'Wife!' I said.

His blue eyes lit up and then became teary. 'Yes, that's Maureen, and she's been a champion through this. I don't know what I would do without her.'

I nodded. I felt so sorry for him. To have a leg amputated! I couldn't imagine how hard that would be.

I suddenly felt lucky. After all, I hadn't had a leg chopped off. I still had the opportunity to learn to walk again.

Sitting there with Steve made me think of a quote I had often heard my father use when I was growing up: 'I cried because I had no shoes, until I met a man who had no feet.'

Since my father's death from pneumonia in 2010, which was three years after my stroke, I've often wondered who first came up with those lines.[1] Whatever the case, I guess Dad used those lines to remind people to be thankful for what they have instead of complaining about what they lack.

And what I had was both my legs. Sitting there with Steve, I felt blessed.

Other Stroke Survivors

Any time someone was admitted to rehab because of a stroke, I felt I had to meet that person straight away. I was always so curious!

I remember one stroke survivor in particular. He was about fifty-five years old and very thin. One of the nursing staff told me he was a big drinker. She said that heavy drinking raises the blood pressure, and that high blood pressure is a big risk factor for stroke.

This man couldn't talk. I wanted to help.

I noticed he had an abacus, like the ones kids use in primary school. I wondered what the abacus was for. Perhaps for helping him learn to count out loud? With my good hand, I moved the little beads one-by-one along the wire of the wooden frame, counting slowly, 'One, two, three …' But the man never counted with me. In fact, I never heard him speak. After a couple of weeks, I realised there wasn't anything more I could try to do. I had too many problems of my own.

Years later, I saw the abacus man in the street in Ballina. He was drinking and didn't recognise me. It was sad to think he had returned to a lifestyle that was so damaging to his health.

Another stroke survivor I met in rehab was a different story. This man arrived when I was about two months into my stay, right around the time I was starting to regain some movement in my right hand. By this point, I was working on getting my grip correct when holding a large plastic cup. I could confidently stack small wooden blocks on top of each other, and I was having a type of electrical muscle stimulation, or EMS.

For the EMS, Lisa would attach electrodes to my right hand. These channelled electrical impulses into my nerves and muscles, helping to make them stronger. At the same time, I was also still doing the worksheets Narelle liked giving me, especially the ones that required me to write the letters of the alphabet in giant letters. I wasn't very good at filling in those worksheets, but pressed on with high hopes.

So that's where I was at when I met this new fellow, who told me he had suffered a stroke many years earlier. He came across as eccentric and a bit pompous, but as I'd discovered from getting to know people like Edith and the old Chinese woman, it's possible to find something to like about even the most difficult personalities – especially once you come to know more about them and the challenges they face.

Anyway, I liked this new addition to rehab. He read profusely, and I could tell he was intelligent. He had his left arm in a sling and had checked himself into rehab because he was seeking intensive physiotherapy. He was there on a voluntary basis. I admired that.

One day, when this man was having lunch with me, I watched him butter a slice of bread using only one hand. I was fascinated. He took the single slice of bread, and he pressed the knife into the butter, and then somehow he got the butter onto the bread using just his right hand. While doing this, he mentioned that he'd had a stroke on the right side of his brain, which explained why he could use his right hand but not his left, and also why he didn't appear to have any speech difficulties.

Meanwhile, because my stroke had occurred in the left side of my brain, I neglected the right side. So on top of having paralysis on the right side of my body, I was also dealing with a range of symptoms that included having difficulty with speech and language (which I now knew was called 'aphasia'), challenges with object recognition ('agnosia'), and problems with daily activities that previously I'd been able to easily perform ('apraxia'). Added to these symptoms were depression, anxiety, and a tendency to be overwhelmed by emotions.

I remember watching the eccentric man in awe. I hadn't known a person could butter bread with just one hand. *If he can do that with one hand, imagine what I will be able to do one day with two!* I thought. I knew I was lucky and felt confident that I would get my right hand working again, at least to the point where it would be useful in everyday life.

A Cup of Tea and Some Sunshine

At Ballina Rehab, every patient I met had a clear reason to be depressed, some more than others. And even though my physical rehabilitation seemed to be going well – I hadn't had a leg amputated like some of the men with diabetes, nor was I being sent to a nursing home for the final years of my life like Edith – most of the time I still felt very down in the dumps.

One afternoon I felt particularly depressed, like I was trapped in a nightmare and couldn't see a way out.

I was sitting on my bed having a good cry when one of the

centre's social workers came by. An Irish-born woman close to retirement age, Helen was actually a woman I knew fairly well on a personal level. We'd sung together in the Voices in the Roar choir, and even though I thought she was a superb person, I still had trouble talking with her about how sad I was feeling.

Our conversation started out as follows.

Helen: How are you today?

Me: Yes.

Helen: How are you feeling?

Me: No. No good.

Helen: You've had a stroke, Jenny. That takes some getting used to. What you're feeling is quite normal.

Helen could see I was in a deep depression. As I began to sob, she dropped the idea of having our usual conversation and sat beside me on the bed. She put an arm around my shoulders while I bawled. Eventually, she fetched my tissue box and handed it to me. I began to quieten down.

'There, that's better,' she said. 'It does you good to have a big cry.'

It took all my energy to utter one word: 'Hopeless.' Then I started crying again.

When finally I couldn't cry anymore, I tried to put on a brave face. 'Yes,' I said, shortly followed by, 'No.' My usual repertoire of words.

Once again, Helen put a reassuring arm around me. 'You've had a stroke, Jenny. That takes some time to get used to.'

I nodded.

'In this situation, what you're feeling is quite normal,' she explained.

'Yes, yes,' I said, in a tone of resignation.

Helen continued speaking in a calm voice. 'Jenny, I think you should talk to your doctor about taking antidepressants.'

'No, no, no, no, no!'

Helen persisted. 'They really can do some good.'

'No!'

Helen kept her arm around me. 'You'll only need a low dose, Jenny. You can start slow and gradually you'll find yourself feeling cheerful again.'

I listened.

'Can you at least think about it?' Helen asked.

'Yes,' I said, somewhat begrudgingly.

I liked Helen's next suggestion a lot better. 'What about a cup of tea and some sunshine?'

I smiled. Just a little. 'Yes, please.'

Helen and I went to the dining room for a cup of tea.

A Light in My Brain

I didn't want to take antidepressants – taking them felt like giving in, like opting for the easy way out – but I followed Helen's suggestion and talked to a doctor about them. I also had to be honest with myself; I needed them.

Over the following few weeks, as the medication kicked in, I began to feel better. My overall confidence returned and I started to feel less anxious. Ultimately, I was grateful to Helen for pushing me towards antidepressants at my greatest time of need.

Ten years later, at the time of writing this book, I've had periods where things have been going so smoothly that I've decided I don't need the antidepressants any more. I go off them for a while, but then the moment I encounter any difficulties in life, like a romantic relationship going haywire, I sink into utter despair.

As this has happened a few times, I've realised that I'll probably need to stay on antidepressants indefinitely. Since having the stroke, I need them. They've been a lifesaver. I feel that there's something in them that puts a light in my brain so that I can function again.

Visitors

While in rehab I had a lot of visitors. This was a blessing as I was in rehab for two and a half months, which sometimes felt like a lifetime.

One of my first visitors was a fellow teacher who turned up only the day after my admission. When he arrived it was just after dinner. He said he was representing the Lismore Teachers Association, and he gave me flowers and a card signed by all my colleagues. I remember he was shocked to see me. I must have looked like a vegetable, as at that stage I wasn't really speaking or moving very much at all. There was such a look of horror on his face. He gave me the flowers and the card, and made a quick exit. I couldn't blame him.

From that point, the visitors just kept coming. There were a lot of teachers. My head teacher, Dot Huey, came every three days. She was a music teacher who would sometimes take me on walks in the grounds. I liked the way she didn't ask me what she could do to help; she just thought of something and did it. I really looked forward to those walks. Dot was so kind, and it was lovely to get out into the fresh air. I also had visits from art teachers, a science teacher who used to be a vet, and a physical education teacher who was interested in the gym.

One of my most frequent visitors was Jane, my loving friend who lived in Ballina. Not only did Jane come to see me in rehab, where she would help me with tasks like putting on my nightie, but on numerous occasions she also took me back to her place for dinner. I would sit in her lounge room with her partner Simon watching reruns of *The Simpsons*. I liked the sense of normality. I would have a glass of wine and relax and feel almost normal. One time I was enjoying myself so much at Jane's that I completely lost track of the time. When Jane got me back to rehab the door was locked, so I had to get back into rehab via the maze of corridors in Ballina District Hospital. I am forever grateful to Jane for all her patience and kindness during that time.

Visitors from further afield included Dad's cousin Raymond and his wife Janece, who came all the way from Sydney. Ray had been for many years the principal of Fairfield High School, where I'd also worked for almost ten years. Ray and Janece talked about what their children were up to and gave me a beautiful shawl. The shawl, decorated with small hand-embroidered butterflies, was very pretty and lifted my spirits.

Another memorable visit occurred the day I came back from swimming with Lisa to find my room full of familiar faces. I saw my Aunty June, my older cousin Bruce and his wife

Michelle, and their daughter Phoebe. This was the Bruce who, back when he was a toddler, had given our grandfather the name 'Bamps' because he couldn't pronounce 'Gramps' – and the name had stuck. Bruce was now a doctor in Sydney, and I was besotted with his daughter, Little Phoebe, who was only about twelve months old.

Within minutes, I was nursing Phoebe on my knee because I could do that. As I was goo-goo-ing and gaa-gaa-ing over her, Brad turned up with our puppy Millie, who was only a couple of months old at the time. Remember earlier in this book I mentioned that Brad and I had adopted Uncle Alfie's dog, a Cavalier King Charles Spaniel named Splat? Well, Splat was like a substitute child for me, so I cried buckets of tears when she died in 2006. Anyway, Brad knew how much I loved her, and while I was in rehab he bought me another Cavalier King Charles Spaniel – and this was Millie, who was now running around the room making Phoebe laugh so much.

Millie was allowed into rehab because the nurses turned a blind eye, which was nice. This beautiful tan and white dog always lifted my spirits – and had done so since the moment I had met her. Since my stroke my memory is not good, but I can recall in vivid detail the day she came into my life. I remember I was home on weekend release from Ballina Rehab, and while Jane was visiting Brad said he'd just duck out to deliver some worm farms, but in reality he was at the airport picking up a puppy he had ordered from an interstate breeder of Cavalier Kings Charles Spaniels! When he walked into the house with the puppy, I knew in a heartbeat that I would call her Millie after the toy dog Dad had given me a few weeks earlier.

Anyway, the day of the visit of the family to my rehab room, Brad was on his best behaviour. He was being the life of the party, trying to get Phoebe to pat the dog. Phoebe was curious about Millie so she attempted to pat her, but Millie was too quick for her. Millie wriggled out of Brad's grip, jumped down to the floor and got away.

Phoebe looked at the dog with surprise but just kept sitting on my knee while Brad was chasing Millie around.

'Never mind,' he eventually said.

It was at that moment that one of the kitchen staff members brought us all some afternoon tea. Madeira cake and muffins! I was very hungry from all the exertion of swimming and socialising, so I was happy to see the food! Too soon the visit was over. I waved everyone goodbye.

Not long after the lively visit from Bruce and his family, Mum and Dad told me I was going to have another very special visitor: my brother John. I was so excited at the thought of seeing John, who was coming all the way from Darwin. First, John had to fly from Darwin to Brisbane, and once he was in Brisbane he would hire a car and drive down to Ballina. My parents had arranged for us to meet him in a restaurant that was within walking distance of the hospital. I walked there with Brad and my parents, being very cautious along the way. Although I had just gotten rid of my cane, I still had my arm in a sling. I didn't want to fall.

We arrived at the restaurant and waited for John. I was getting impatient. I still couldn't say little more than, 'Yes. No. I don't think so.' I sat silently. Waiting.

John arrived. I got to my feet quickly and felt all my love

for my little brother surge through me. I wanted to cry. I tried not to cry. I wanted to talk to John but I couldn't and that was so frustrating. I burst into tears.

My little brother hugged me and it suddenly seemed as if everything would be all right. Because John was the youngest child in our family, our nickname for him was Min, which was short for Mini – and we still called him that even though he had grown into a big strong man. Dad was hugging him and saying, 'Min! My boy! My boy!' John kissed Mum, saying that his wife Kirsty had asked him to send her love to everyone. By then I was sitting back down, just watching John. It felt so good to see him.

We ordered our meals and I didn't pay much attention to the process. Brad was being congenial and that was good. The meal came. I had chicken scaloppine. It smelt nice but I couldn't cut the meat with one hand. So Mum automatically reached over and cut it for me. Then she attempted to feed me. I said firmly, 'No. No.' I refused to eat my food when Mum was trying to feed me.

'I don't think so!' I snapped.

Picking up my fork in my left hand, I started stabbing at the portions of food that Mum had cut for me. I was really making my displeasure felt.

The atmosphere was uncomfortable.

Brad eventually said, 'Enough of that.'

I started feeling sorry about my behaviour, but didn't know how to say that.

Mum glossed over it. She said, 'Oh, this is nothing to worry about, Jenny. Isn't it lovely to see your brother!'

Yes, it was lovely to see my brother. I was glad to see John. I felt very loved. He had come all the way from Darwin.

A Brain MRI and a Face like Thunder

At Lismore Base Hospital, I'd had two CT (or 'CAT') scans: one when I was admitted, and another the next day. Years later, I would learn that while a CT scan is usually one of the first tests done in a stroke evaluation (especially in an emergency room), additional testing is often performed at a later stage using magnetic resonance imaging (MRI), which is better at showing soft tissue such as brain tissue. Using magnetic field and radio waves, an MRI scan creates three-dimensional pictures of a body's internal structures. As this type of scan takes longer than a CT scan, it's not usually available under emergency conditions.

Anyway, nineteen days after my stroke, it was time for me to have an MRI. By that stage, my physiotherapy was going really well and I was feeling very proud of the work I'd put into my walking. How ironic, then, that hospital regulations demanded I had to be pushed everywhere in a wheelchair.

A wardsman was given the job of getting me from Ballina Rehab to St Vincent's Private Hospital in Lismore. He was a kind man, and I was pleased he was the one who would be driving me that day – mainly because I thought of him as my friendly neighbourhood breakfast assistant. He was often at work early in the mornings and would pop into my room to open my Weet-Bix packet for me. He was cheery and prepared to venture outside of his basic job description to help out.

But I'm afraid that on that particular day I wasn't respectful of the wardsman's schedule, not to mention the fact that his actions were bound within strict hospital rules. All I knew was that I wanted to walk. I wanted to prove to myself that I was able to.

When the wardsman came to collect me to take me to Lismore, it was lunchtime. I was in the dining room having a sandwich. I knew it was time for me to go for my MRI, and when I saw him approaching me with a wheelchair, I stood up saying, 'Walk! Walk!' and scurried out into the lobby.

The warden followed me, still pushing the wheelchair. 'I know you can walk, Jenny,' he said gently, 'but you need to get into the wheelchair. We have rules.'

I stubbornly refused to sit in the wheelchair, so he continued, 'It's for your own safety, Jenny. What if you fell and ended up with a broken arm or leg?'

I could see a pleading look in his eyes. Finally, with bad grace, I got into the wheelchair, and he pushed me to the minibus.

During the half-hour drive from the rehab unit to St Vincent's, I didn't say a word to the poor wardsman. I even cursed him under my breath.

When we arrived at St Vincent's, I was still giving him the silent treatment. He was probably relieved to hand me over to the nurse who wheeled me to the radiology department. Everyone there could see I had a face like thunder.

The MRI scanner was in a large room divided by a glass partition, and there were two men sitting behind the glass. They tried to jolly me along, and I finally got over my bad mood.

'I'm Brett, and this is Colin,' one of the men said. 'You're not afraid of confined spaces?'

'No,' I said.

'Great,' Brett continued. 'The space where you'll be lying is small and you'll have to be very still. We're going to have a look at your brain using MRI.'

I stared through the glass partition at the MRI machine, which appeared to be a large white cylinder. Brett explained that I would lie on a table, and that the table would then slide into the mouth of the cylinder. The whole set-up looked impressive.

It was time for me to get ready for my scan. Colin said, 'Do you need help getting out of the wheelchair?'

This was my chance to be independent. I was going to prove I could walk. I took a deep breath and stood up by myself, and then I walked with a nurse to a curtained cubicle. The nurse helped me undress and put on a cotton gown. She took off my watch and jewellery. Then it was time for me to hop onto the table, go into the machine, and have my scan.

Colin had told me the scan would take about an hour, and even though the machine was making a lot of noises that sounded like knocks, loud bangs and clicks, I dozed through most of the procedure.

The same wardsman from Ballina drove me back to rehab. I was relieved to have the scan over and done with, and now felt guilty about my earlier behaviour. I wanted to make it up to him. I said sorry, and he said, 'That's all right', and I felt cheerful again.

I gazed out the minibus window and thought how silly I'd

been. I knew I could walk and I also knew that the rehab unit and hospital had policies and were right to stick with them. I chastised myself, saying quietly under my breath, 'What will be, will be.'

As we drove down the cutting from the Alstonville plateau towards Ballina, with the welcome blue of the Pacific Ocean spreading out before us, I thought again of all the times the wardsman had kindly opened my Weet-Bix packets, even though Narelle had told me to do it myself. I remember one day he was about to do it for me when Narelle appeared in my room. 'No, I want Jenny to do it on her own.' But as soon as Narelle had gone, the wardsman had given me a wink and opened the packet anyway.

The minibus pulled up outside the rehab centre. As the wardsman helped me out of the vehicle, I gave him the biggest smile I could muster. In my mind, I told myself I would become a better person.

MRI Results

Once back at Ballina Rehab, I realised how relieved I was to have the MRI over and done with. I relaxed, not worrying at all about what the results would be. Instead, I looked forward to my next round of speech therapy sessions with Rose. What did she have in store for me?

After only a fortnight of speech therapy, I could say many more words than my original 'Yes', 'No' and 'I don't think so'. Some of my new words were 'coffee', 'sandwich', and 'toilet'. Rose was proud of me, but she also wanted me to keep working. A few days after the MRI, she reminded me I was still having trouble speaking in sentences and urged me to keep practising.

I had no problem with that. Only the day before, I'd been busting for a wee. I needed a nurse to help me. Seeing one pass by, I caught her attention with one of my new words: 'Toilet.'

'I'll only be a jiffy,' the nurse said, scurrying off to another patient's room.

A few minutes later, I saw her walk by again. I repeated the word, this time quite loudly. 'Toilet! Toilet!'

But by the time the nurse finally came to help me, I had wet my pants. I started to cry. 'Messy mess,' I said, feeling ashamed of myself.

Now, in the speech therapy room with Rose, I wondered if that humiliating episode could have been avoided if I had been able to say, 'Nurse! I am about to wet my pants. I need a toilet now, this very minute!'

'Your speech is much clearer, Jenny,' Rose explained, breaking into my thoughts. 'But it's still what I'd describe as *telegraphic*. This means it's a bit like a telegram – abbreviated, with some filler words missing.'

To help me speak more fluently, Rose showed me a game that began with a sequence of illustrated cards. She held up the first one. 'What's this?' she asked.

'Girl,' I said.

'Good. And this?' She raised another card, and I saw the same girl standing in a shop, admiring some dresses.

'Shopping,' I said.

'Yes,' Rose said. 'The girl is shopping. And how does she feel?'

'Happy.'

'What's she buying?' Rose asked.

'Graduation dress,' I said promptly.

'Very good!' Rose nodded. 'Now we have to run everything together, as in: The girl is happy that she is buying a graduation dress. You try.'

On the table in front of us, she fanned out a second sequence of cards.

'Boy,' I said in response to the first card. Then, 'Sweets.'

'Now run it all together,' Rose instructed.

'Boy buys sweets,' I said.

'Yes,' Rose agreed. 'And what about his emotions?'

'Joyful!'

'Okay. Run the words together.'

'Boy joyfully buys sweets!' I was getting the hang of this.

Rose gave me a lovely smile. 'Excellent work, Jenny!'

Apparently this is what I was doing – thinking about girls shopping for dresses and boys buying sweets – on the very afternoon that someone in Lismore was giving my parents and Brad the results from my MRI scan. Perhaps this 'someone' was a specialist in acute stroke care, or possibly even a neurologist; I have no idea, and my mother can't remember. But the upshot was that the results confirmed what the initial CAT scans had suggested: that in my brain's left hemisphere, I had suffered a stroke 'through the basal ganglia to the cerebral cortex of the posterior frontal lobe'.

Although this was not good information in anyone's book, the MRI had also revealed some happier news. Apart from the stroke, there were no other causes for my symptoms. The scan had not found a brain tumour, for example, and my artery supply was 'now entirely within normal limits'. There was no sign of any aneurysms that could kill me if they burst.

Many years later, I would wonder if the Cyklokapron and Triphasil tablets I had been taking to reduce my heavy bleeding could have been contributing factors to my stroke. Occasionally, I've asked GPs about this, and one admitted that both drugs 'could have the kind of effect that would increase the possibility of clotting and thus the stroke', but that 'this effect would be in conjunction with my own natural increased chance of suffering a stroke'.

In other words, the doctor quoted above, like many other medicos, said it wasn't possible to pin down the cause of my stroke.

But one day a friend researched the severe medical warnings associated with taking both drugs together, and learnt that: 'These medicines may interact and cause very harmful effects and are usually not taken together ... Both of these medicines can increase your risk of a blood clot.'

If I hadn't been taking these drugs would I have had the stroke? I'll never know.

The Weekly Conference

Mostly, I kept my head down and concentrated on getting well. Once a week, though, I had to listen to medical discussions.

Ballina Rehab held case conferences every Wednesday morning. This was when the doctors, physiotherapists, speech therapists and occupational therapists talked about the progress of the patients. After the conference, every patient had his or her own appointment with the disability and rehabilitation specialist, a lovely man named Dr Harry Franklin.

Dr Franklin was an older person with a pleasant bedside manner; I felt he was someone who could help me. My parents or Brad usually took me to these appointments, but one day I went alone. Dr Franklin had a medical student with him.

Looking at me kindly, Dr Franklin asked, 'Jenny, do I have your permission to talk about your situation?' He gave me an encouraging smile and waited for me to nod before continuing. 'This is Michael, he's studying medicine and he wants to find out about you and see how he can help.'

Michael was looking directly at me. He said hello.

After explaining to Michael that I had aphasia, Dr Franklin gently manipulated my right arm in an upwards direction, saying, 'It's amazing the progress Jenny is making. After her left CVA on June 8, she was frozen on the right side.'

He then turned to me. 'What do you think of your progress, Jenny?'

With difficulty, I said, 'Mmm, good. Words hard. Arm moves … happy.'

I wanted to discuss more complex things, but speaking in sentences was difficult without Rose there. With Rose, I could take my time. I didn't have to rush.

'Walk around and show Michael how well you're doing,' the doctor suggested.

I walked around the office. Both men smiled. Then Michael examined my right arm and did the standard series of physical tests, taking more time than Dr Franklin normally would. He checked my knee-jerk reflexes and my blood pressure, which were fine. He seemed confident and shy, all at the same time.

As Michael did his tests, I thought of my father and my youngest brother. Dad was a gynaecologist, and Mark had worked as the Senior Registrar in Psychiatry at Alice Springs. I thought of how Dad and Mark, when learning about medicine, would have found themselves in situations like this: learning under supervision while working with real patients.

Thinking of Mark, I felt like crying.

My parents had three children. First, there was me, born in 1962. Twenty months later, my brother Mark came into the world. A few years after that, Mark and I welcomed our little brother John. I grew up to be a high school teacher, John became a lawyer who is now the Senior Manager of Investment Opportunities at Indigenous Business Australia, and Mark followed his passion for psychiatry to Alice Springs, where he became devoted to the welfare of indigenous people in remote communities. For his PhD, Mark carried out a lot of original research on how to help the traditional owners of this land.

But my beautiful brother Mark was only thirty-three when he died of bowel cancer. This happened in 1998. On the first anniversary of his death, the Remote Mental Health Service in Alice Springs was renamed in his honour, and is now called the Dr Mark Sheldon Remote Mental Health Service. I was proud of my brother's achievements, and so completely heartbroken that he had died – not just because he was my brother, but also because as a compassionate young psychiatrist he was already making such a difference in the world.

I couldn't help thinking that if Mark were still alive he would step into this situation with my stroke and take control. I suddenly missed him so much. As Michael continued his assessment, I thought back to a dream I'd had when Mark was first ill. In the dream, we were on a car racecourse. We got into the back of a car together. A professional racing driver was driving the car, and we were racing along at top speed when Mark fell out. I wanted to go back for him but couldn't get the driver to stop. I woke up from the dream and that was when I knew Mark was going to die.

Michael must have sensed that I was upset. He stopped what he was doing and asked if I was okay. I smiled and said, 'Yes, no, I don't know.'

The young man looked worried, so I tried harder to make him feel okay. 'Yes, yes!' I managed to say. I wanted to be a good patient for this student doctor. I wanted to help. I felt closer to my brother that way.

Pretty Baby

You might remember Helen Flanagan from an earlier part of my story? Well, Helen was not the only social worker I knew. There was also Margot Henry, who worked at the Carroll Centre, which was a day rehabilitation centre at St Vincent's Private Hospital in Lismore. Apart from being social workers, Helen and Margot had something else in common; they were both in a choir called Voices in the Roar, which is a choir I had also belonged to before having my stroke.

One afternoon I was lying in bed feeling very sorry for

myself. It was only 4pm, but already I wanted to just go to sleep and forget about the world. This is when Margot walked into my room for a visit, and along with Margot came Kathleen Mills, another choir friend. I was so happy to see them!

'How are you getting along?' Kathleen asked.

'Yes,' I said, because I couldn't say anything else. Then I started to cry.

This is when Kathleen mentioned she was a speech therapist, just like Rose. I was so surprised; I hadn't known that was Kathleen's job!

Margot handed me a box of tissues. I hadn't realised I was crying. As I wiped my face, I tried explaining my frustration about how hard it was to communicate. The fact it was so hard to express my frustration only made me more frustrated. I started to cry again. Those tissues sure were coming in handy.

Kathleen said that next time she visited she'd bring her computer. She said there was a program on it that could help me to communicate.

Sure enough, the next time Margot and Kathleen came to see me, Kathleen had her laptop with her. On the laptop was a program with a long name that began with 'P'. It was a symbol-based application that gives voice to people who can't speak, and also helps with language skills and development. If I touched a picture of an apple, for example, a voice would say 'apple'. But I found I had so much to say – and my vocabulary was so extensive – that the pictures just couldn't express my thoughts.

For weeks, I had been working so hard to communicate with everyone using only the few words I could say – still little more than: 'yes', 'no' and 'I don't think so'. This situation relied on people asking me the right questions so I could make true and logical statements. Otherwise, I was lost. To everyone around me, it probably looked like I didn't know what I wanted to say, but I did know! The words were inside my head; they just wouldn't come out.

Facial expressions gave me a whole extra vocabulary I could draw on, especially as I had done drama training and for many years had practiced getting feelings onto my face for others to read. This skill was still there for me. I hate to think how I would have coped without it.

But during my time at rehab, I rarely felt that a few words and my facial expressions were enough. And now, even with a computerised language program in front of me, I still didn't have enough tools at my disposal. This program really wasn't for me.

'No, no,' I said to Kathleen after an hour of trying to work with it.

Kathleen was very good about the situation. Packing up her laptop, she graciously told me, 'It was worth a try, Jenny. You have so much to say. I guess this program is just too simple.'

Again, I was crying. And again, Margot and Kathleen were looking at me with concern. I could feel them trying to think of something that would make me feel better.

Finally, Margot said, 'What about if Voices in the Roar come and sing here?

I was so excited. The joy on my face spoke volumes. I said, 'Yes, yes, yes, yes!'

Kathleen said, 'Then we'll do it. I'll contact the others, and we will come. We'll make it one evening at around seven o'clock, so that choir members who work can get here.'

That night in bed, I realised I was happy. Singing always felt so good to me that even the thought of singing made me cheerful! And I knew I'd be able to join in with the choir. After all, even though I couldn't talk properly, I was able to sing. I had my iPod with me in rehab. The iPod had all my favourite songs on it, and I loved to sing along as I listened to them. Sometimes, it felt like the music was the only thing keeping me sane.

Even though I didn't know it at the time, research has shown that many people with non-fluent aphasia can sing fluently. The Swedish physician Olaf Dalin first reported it in 1736. This was after he saw a young man who had lost his ability to speak following a brain injury suddenly start singing hymns. Today, many therapists working with aphasic patients have witnessed this same seemingly impossible feat. Mostly it happens with people like me who have lost spoken communication skills after having a left-sided stroke.

You see, the left hemisphere of the brain is mainly responsible for processing language, so someone with a left-hemisphere stroke is more likely to experience aphasia. On the other hand, singing uses an individual's entire brain, so even someone who cannot speak may be able to tap into other parts of her brain to sing instead.

But regardless of what brain science says, I know singing is good for me.

Music was the spoonful of sugar that kept me going in

rehab, and I didn't need scientific research and MRI scans to tell me that.

I had always loved to sing! I especially adored all the old musicals featuring Fred Astaire and Ginger Rogers. As a little girl of six or seven, I was crazy about movies with titles like *The Gay Divorcee* and *The Barkleys of Broadway*.

At around this age, I was staying at my grandparents' house in Bardwell Park in Sydney. My family had just moved up from the South Coast of NSW, and while Mum and Dad were looking for a house for us, I was watching *Pretty Baby* on the television. Afterwards, I kept humming the theme song.

My grandfather 'Bamps' wasn't just a wonderful grandfather, he was also a self-taught piano player who composed many brilliant songs.

I wanted to hear Bamps play the *Pretty Baby* song. He had a grand piano. I never considered playing the instrument without his permission. Even though I was his favourite grandchild, it would've been more than my life was worth. So I went and found Bamps in his office. I knew he could play anything by ear, so I hummed him the tune. Bamps led me straight into the living room and sat in front of his pride and joy. As he played, I sang along.

'Everybody loves a baby, that's why I'm in love with you. Pretty baby. Pretty baby. And I'd like to be your sister, brother, dad and mother too. Pretty baby. Pretty baby!'

I decided I was going to be a singer and an actor. I also had my heart set on becoming a dancer – despite the fact I had 'two left feet'. It's no surprise that as an adult I became involved with various choirs in Sydney – such as the Stay Tuned choir in Glebe.

But one of my favourite choirs was called Stairwell to Heaven. And yes, I mean 'stairwell' (as in the part of a building where a staircase is located), rather than 'stairway' (a flight of steps that actually gets you somewhere). This was because in the beginning all the choir's rehearsals were held in a stairwell.

Stuart Davis was the director of this choir, which rehearsed at Annandale Primary School. Stuart's children attended the school, and he'd started the choir a few years earlier at the urging of parents. Three years later, the choir would perform at my wedding. It was a good choir.

At around the age of thirty, I'd begun to follow my dream of becoming a jazz singer. I felt it was my destiny. *You only live once; you have to do what you want!* I thought. So I took leave from my full-time teaching job at Marist Sisters' College in Woolwich, where I'd been working for five years, and signed up for casual teaching work at St Scholastica's College in Glebe, which was a lot closer to where I was living at the time. Later, I would also accept a casual position at Fairfield High School, which would eventually lead to a permanent teaching position that I would hold for around ten years … which I guess signals that I never did manage to forge a full-time career as a professional jazz singer.

But I did have fun trying!

Fly Me to the Moon

I began my quest to be a professional jazz singer by going to

Kate Dunbar's 'Jazz Singers Workshop', which was held every week at the Strawberry Hills Hotel in Surry Hills. This workshop provided me with an opportunity to perform with a jazz quartet, improve my performance, meet other jazz singers and have fun. Kate created a very safe and friendly environment, so when I got things wrong I didn't feel embarrassed. It was a great place to learn. I went to several workshops and struck up a friendship with the pianist there. What a pity I can't remember his name. He was an elderly man and a real charmer, and couldn't he tinkle the ivories!

At one time at the workshop I was singing a song called *Embraceable You*, and I was experimenting with singing it slowly until reaching the bridge, and then singing it fast. It was a workshop, after all. 'Come to mama, come to mama do,' I sang, 'my sweet embraceable you!' At the end, I couldn't wait to hear the critique from Kate, but for some reason she moved on to the next person without commenting on my performance. I was very frustrated. I had come along for feedback.

After the workshop, the elderly pianist complimented me on the song and offered a suggestion that would make a huge difference to my life. He advised me to go to Freddie Wilson. I had no idea who Freddie Wilson was, but I agreed to go.

I met this Freddie Wilson at his house, which was an ordinary house in Hunters Hill. Freddie's wife Bev greeted me at the door and invited me in for coffee. Then Freddie walked into the room. He was a slight man and I sensed he wouldn't take fools lightly. I was a bit afraid. But also intrigued.

By that stage, I knew that Freddie was a fabulous jazz musician, and that twice a week he ran two jazz classes: one for musicians who wanted to play jazz on instruments such as the saxophone, trumpet, trombone, piano, double bass, drums and guitar; and the other for singers who wanted to sing jazz. I didn't have much idea of what to expect, but felt I was in the right place.

The sessions were held in a garage at the back of Freddie and Bev's house. At the first session I went to, there were eight singers as well as a drummer, a double bass player and a piano player. Freddie would scribble out chords for singers on pieces of paper, and everyone was allowed to sing two songs. Freddie was mentoring a singer called Geoff, who was a real crooner – not to mention handsome, tall, blonde and blue-eyed. Geoff got up to sing first and boy could he sing. I wanted to be like him!

The first song I performed was *Ain't Misbehavin'*. 'I don't stay out late, don't care to go,' I sang. 'I'm home about eight, just me and my radio. Ain't misbehavin'. I'm savin' my love for you.' I'd chosen that song because my father played it on the piano, and it was a favourite of mine. The feedback Freddie gave me was blunt and hilarious, and it was also encouraging and detailed. It was feedback I could work with. I felt ready to do my second song.

This second song was 'Oh What a Little Moonlight Can Do'. I had trouble counting in, which wasn't unusual for me, but soon found myself being carried along by the rapid tempo. 'Ooh, ooh, ooh. What a little moonlight can do. Ooh, ooh ooh. What a little moonlight can do to you.'

I liked Billie Holiday's version best and tried to phrase the lyrics the way she did when she first recorded the song in

1935. 'You're in love. Your heart's a-flutter ... and all day long ... you only stutter ... cos your poor tongue ... just won't utter the words ... I love you!'

When I finished singing, Freddie was highly critical. But this didn't bother me, as a lot of people had told me that high praise from Freddie was rare. Freddie made me sing it over again, straight away. He knew I wanted to deliver it quickly, the way Billie Holiday did, so he recommended that I 'talk slowly to make it quicker'. I know that seems counterintuitive, but it works! Taking Freddie's advice on board and singing the song again was a pivotal moment. It took me a while to get the hang of that particular technique, but the effort was worth it.

Anyway, from that moment I was hooked. I went to Freddie's sessions twice a week: one on a weeknight and the other on a Saturday morning. After a few weeks of these sessions with Freddie, we celebrated everything we'd learnt by holding a special concert. One night some of us also sang at a jazz club in George Street that no longer exists.

Freddie, sadly, is in the same boat. He was such a character. He was sometimes cranky and downright cantankerous. And I liked him. He was a good person. But he smoked, and that was what killed him in the end.

Around the time of these Freddie sessions, I was also learning a lot from a pianist called Paul Haire, who was wonderful to me – having me over to his place to practice, and writing chord charts for me and generally becoming my mentor. I'd met Paul during an organised tour of Europe in the late 1990s. The tour had begun in England, and had then taken us through

Italy, Munich, Switzerland and Paris, before ending back in England. There were about eighteen of us on the tour, but Paul was the person I instantly hit it off with – mainly over our love of music. He was a jazz pianist and he'd studied at the Sydney Conservatorium of Music.

Paul wore goggle-like glasses and needed to stay out of the sun because he was an albino man. There was a dreadful girl on our tour who kept teasing him for wearing such unusual glasses. I felt sorry for him so I stuck up for him. One day when she'd been teasing him, we went back to the hotel where we were staying and he played the piano, and it was like all his emotions came out in the music. I was impressed. Once we were back home in Australia he rang me up and we kept our friendship going.

Anyway, with help from Paul and Freddy, I began singing at other people's gigs … and the more I sang at other people's gigs, the more I wanted to get my own. Finally, the moment arrived!

I managed to get a gig at the Exchange Hotel in Balmain on Monday nights. I had to get an ABN number – so officially, I was a professional jazz singer! I organised for Paul to provide piano accompaniment, and we were successful. The night was billed as a 'jazz jam', which meant that other people could get up and sing too. Paul and I had an understanding; he was doing a lot of the leading and he needed to. I was very grateful to him.

Over the following months, I sometimes suspected Paul was a little in love with me but I ignored that because in those days I always went for the unsuitable types. Later I was interested in Brad Miller and that was that. Anyway, Paul Haire and I established a good working relationship, picking up quite a few gigs together. There was a wedding at the HMAS Penguin Royal Australian Navy Base at Balmoral on Sydney Harbour's Middle Head, and that was nice. But my favourite performance with Paul was actually our first one, and I often reminisce about it.

The date was sometime early in 2002. I remember walking to the microphone stand at the Exchange Hotel and looking out across the pub. The hotel patrons were noisy and didn't appear to be in any hurry to give me their full attention. I saw women chatting in small groups, men laughing together, and bar staff wandering about picking up glasses. I felt determined to change this.

The percussion instruments and the guitar and the piano all were playing an introductory instrumental piece. I was nervous. I braced myself. Then I was introduced and the next thing I knew I was addressing the patrons. 'This is Jazz Jam and I'm Jenny Sheldon. I'm going to sing a few numbers straight up for you now, but for anyone else who wants to sing, all you have to do is see Melanie … ' I gestured towards another singer, who waved to the audience so everyone would know who she was. 'And now, let's dive into our first set with a song you'll all know: *Fly Me To The Moon*. Okay boys, count me in …'

Singing this particular number always made me feel so happy!

'Fly me to the moon and let me play among the stars. Let me see what spring is like on Jupiter and Mars.'

The lyrics really express the soaring feeling people have when they're falling in love!

'In other words, hold my hand. In other words, darling, kiss me.'

I always try to sing this number in a classical and uplifting way, swinging my delivery on the bridge.

'Fill my heart with song and let me sing for evermore. You are all I long for, all I worship and adore.'

And I like to sing the final two lyrics three times in a row!

'In other words, please be true. In other words, I love you.'

Singing gave me a natural high, and I wanted to do it more and more. I loved singing all the classic jazz songs. That night I also sang *Blue Moon*, *I Got a Crush on You*, *God Bless the Child*, *They Can't Take That Away from Me*, and *It Had to Be You*. When I stopped to take a break, there were plenty of people to talk to about the performance, and there were lots of other willing singers.

The band and I did three sets that night, and in between our sets I got to introduce the other singers. I really was having a ball.

But suddenly, while singing a song called *Wave* during our final set, an actual wave of sadness washed over me. I began thinking of my brother Mark who had died, and I sang the rest of the song like there was no tomorrow. The words came straight from my heart: 'So close your eyes, for that's a lovely way to be. Aware of things your heart alone was meant to see. The fundamental loneliness goes whenever two can dream a dream together.'

The poignancy of my delivery must have come through to the audience, as the applause at the end of that song was deafening. They had liked it. That song was definitely the highlight of the night.

The Power of Song

Memories of my performances at the Jazz Jam nights often kept me going as I worked hard in rehab to strengthen my arm's muscles or practice holding a plastic cup. But none of my daydreams came close to the real thing: to singing with others, or singing with others *for* others. So bless Kathleen for keeping her promise. The week after she had last visited with Margot, I was sitting having lunch one day when a nurse came up and sat at the table beside me.

'Jenny, I have some news for you,' she said, leaning forward with her elbows on the table so she could smile right into my face. I got the feeling she was waiting to see me smile back.

'Yes,' I said, already starting to grin.

'Your Voices in the Roar choir will be here tomorrow night at seven o'clock!'

The joy on my face!

The nurse laughed to see it and walked happily off to resume her duties as I tucked back into my food.

Excitement! I was finally going to sing with my choir.

The next night, ten of the choir members came to Ballina Rehab. Everyone had assembled by seven o'clock: four men and six women, including Helen the social worker, and Margot and Kathleen. I hugged everyone!

Quite a few patients and various staff members had gathered in a little courtyard to hear our concert, as the TV was on in the dining room. First we sang *That Lonesome Road* by James Taylor. 'Walk down that lonesome road all by yourself. Don't turn your head back over your shoulder, and only stop to rest yourself when the silver moon is shining high above the trees.'

Someone had brought a guitar along, which sounded lovely when we sang *Lean on Me*. Then everyone asked me if there was anything special I wanted to sing. Without hesitation I said *Edelweiss*. We began singing *Edelweiss* – 'Eldeweiss, edelweiss, ev'ry morning you greet me …' – and I could get out every word! 'Small and white, clean and bright, you look happy to meet me.'

The patients and staff in rehab loved the music. They were humming along to it. After the choir had finished singing outside, we wandered down the hallways to visit individual wards. Some patients didn't want to be disturbed because they were too sick, but others were happy for us to come and sing for them. The nurses thought the singing was great, and one announced to the choir members, 'You can come any time!'

And a couple of weeks later, the choir did come again. And for a second time, we had a wonderful concert. I was so grateful to *Voices in the Roar*, as singing with them was the most amazing thing that happened while I was there. As Kathleen would write to me in an email several years later, 'Visiting you was something that the choir loved. We could see the happiness that singing gave you, the freedom of the words flowing with no restraint at last. I thought it was the key to you getting well.'

Questions

When I was still in rehab, some of the staff did an assessment of my house and suggested some modifications that would need to be carried out before I moved back there. They were concerned that the front step would be dangerous, for example, and I knew that was true; I had already tripped on it during one of my brief visits.

Finally, the house was deemed safe enough for me to spend weekends there. On my first weekend visit, Mum made me lamb cutlets to celebrate.

Usually my weekend visits home began on a Friday. One Friday I was at home when I had a visit from a man from the NSW Department of Education. His name was Martin Boyd. This was when our dog Millie was around. As Martin introduced himself he said, 'Is that your dog out on the road? I'm a bit concerned she'll get hit by a car.'

Brad said, 'Oh, the little bugger!' and went to fetch Millie.

I managed to ask Martin if he'd like a cup of tea or coffee, and as I put the kettle on he made friendly small talk. I could barely say anything else, so I just listened.

Once Brad was back inside, Martin got down to business. He talked a lot and I couldn't follow any of it. All I noticed was that he seemed like a warm and lovely man, and that he was sensitive to my situation. I relied on Brad to understand what Martin was saying. Later, Brad explained that I was currently on full sick pay, but from the following week would only be receiving half of that pay. Eventually, even that half-pay would run out.

The best thing I could do was to focus on getting better. I practiced reading, and soon realised that I could read aloud with little trouble at all. When I was reading, the words came out flowing. It was so maddening that I couldn't do this when speaking!

I became more determined than ever to use the right words when speaking, and to start speaking more fluently. Imagine not being about to think of the right words for a situation – or to know what you want to say and not be able to say it. Often, I could formulate sentences in my mind, but I just couldn't articulate them. So here I was, a school teacher scrambling for words. This situation was all new to me, and I thought back to some of the students I had taught who had had the same problem. At the time, regrettably, I had thought of them as 'not all there'. Now, I was having the same difficulty.

At other times, I had trouble simply coming up with the name of something that I knew well, and in these situations it was hard to try to ask people to help me find the name I was seeking because I couldn't speak in sentences. A clear example of this frustration springs to mind.

One morning, I was walking to the physiotherapy room at Ballina Rehab, and for some reason I was trying to think of the name of a particular book … perhaps because I wanted to read it. It was a book I knew well. I had even taught it at school. The name was on the tip of my tongue. As I entered the room and started doing my exercises with Narelle, I couldn't stop thinking about this matter of the book title.

'Atticus!' I said to Narelle.

Narelle was helping me with some stretches. She looked puzzled.

I got to my feet and pointed to a book that was sitting on a desk. I suddenly felt hopeful. 'Atticus!'

Narelle still looked confused. I kept saying 'Atticus'

while waving the book in front of her face with my left hand. I tend to be an obsessive person. Sometimes this is a good thing and sometimes it's probably annoying for people!

'You're trying to think of the name of a book?' Narelle finally said.

I nodded.

She smiled at me. 'Hmm, I have no idea.'

Damn. But then Lisa walked in. Narelle asked Lisa if she knew of a book that had something to do with the word 'Atticus', but Lisa had no idea either. I tried to put the thought of the book in the back of my mind and continued with my exercises.

I was hoping Mum and Dad would know. I didn't think Brad would have any idea. When the three of them came to visit me later that day I tried again, starting with Dad.

'Atticus!' I said to him.

Dad was interested in what I was trying to say but looked confused and turned to Mum. 'What do you think it is, love?' he asked.

'I don't know!' Mum admitted.

Meanwhile, all I could say was, 'Atticus. Atticus. Atticus.'

Mum could sense my frustration. She gave me a kiss and said, 'I'll think of it, Jenny.'

When my parents and Brad left, I said to the nurses one more time, 'Atticus!' And then I gave up.

A few days later, when I was on leave from rehab for the weekend, I was at Alstonville getting my legs waxed. There was a bookshop next door to the beauty salon. They were bound to have the book I wanted, and I wouldn't even have to know the title. I could just look for it on the shelves!

But I couldn't see the book anywhere. Okay. No problem. Although I couldn't speak well and was worried about that, I would ask the woman at the counter.

I approached the woman and she asked if I'd like some help.

'Atticus!' I said.

She looked at me, perplexed. After a moment, she said, 'Well, I can look up Atticus.'

While the woman was looking at the computer screen, I managed to say, 'Atticus. Don't know author.'

She looked taken aback. I was getting nowhere.

It was time for me to meet Brad, who was coming to pick me up from the beauty salon. When Brad arrived I brought him straight into the bookshop. I was hoping Brad could help me.

But all Brad said was, 'Come on, Jenny. We have to get you back to Ballina Rehab.'

He then turned to the woman. 'Sorry. I don't know what she's saying. She had a stroke.'

'Oh,' the woman said. 'She kept saying "Atticus", but I don't know what that means.'

I must have looked crestfallen. Brad put his arm around me. 'Never mind,' he said. 'You'll think of it later.'

But I didn't think of it later. Imagine how I felt, being a school teacher and knowing the book so well. It wasn't until at least a year later that I finally came across the book in the Lismore Public Library. When I saw it, I grabbed it from the shelf and hugged it tightly to my chest. I'd waited such a long time to read it.

The book was *To Kill a Mockingbird*, the Pulitzer Prize-winning novel by Harper Lee. The novel was known for its warmth, humour and the social conscience of its narrator, the six-year-old Jean Louise Finch, whose nickname is Scout. And the novel's protagonist? Scout's father. Who is a lawyer. And whose name is Atticus Finch.

I thought back to all the times I'd just been saying 'Atticus' into space and expecting everyone to know what I was talking about. Looking back at that time now, I wonder why I didn't just write 'Atticus' on paper and write down a few other words to make my question clearer. But now I know that recovering from a stroke is a long journey. It really is all about taking baby steps.

Progress Report

As I approached my time to leave rehab, Rose reminded me how far I had come.

'You've made significant progress, Jenny,' she said. 'Remember how you could barely speak when you arrived?

I agreed.

'Well, now you're able to follow conversations … not just single words like when you were admitted. You're much less impulsive and this has improved your comprehension. You received multiple speech therapy sessions per day while you were in the rehab unit and you made signficant progress.'

Rose talked about how difficult it is for a right-handed person to learn to write with her left hand. 'This is a very hard thing to do!' she said. 'But you've made great gains in your writing. Even though you had initial difficulties spelling longer words and made consistent errors such as putting letters in the wrong order, you've done lots of practice around your writing, and in developing your "sound to letter" and "letter to sound" conversion system. You also worked on your self-awareness of errors, and now you're writing at a sentence level with minimal errors.'

Of course, Rose said that although my speech was much clearer she would still describe it as 'telegraphic'.

But overall, she was delighted with my progress. 'You've made remarkable gains since your stroke, Jenny,' she said.

I looked up from the worksheet that I was completing.

Rose smiled. 'Look at how well you're writing with your left hand!'

At our final speech therapy session, Rose gave me a list of suggestions for ongoing therapy. These included: documenting daily events; practicing money handling, calculations, computer skills and written expression; answering the phone using a practised script, and then summarising phone calls in writing and jotting down phone numbers; developing intonation and stress in my speech through role playing; explaining picture sequences in words; and reading aloud.

I promised Rose that I would practice those things. I wanted to get well, and if there was one thing that being at Ballina Rehab had taught me, it was that practice definitely counts! I couldn't even sound out the letters of the alphabet at first but I was improving.

Getting Out

Three days before my discharge from Ballina Rehab, Mum and Dad came to my final meeting with Dr Franklin, who praised what he said was the 'amazing' progress I'd made in the previous few months.

But then we were all shocked to hear him say, 'We'll see you back in six months to check how you're going, Jenny, but from this point I'm not sure how much more improvement you'll be able to make.'

My face fell and Dad noticed. He gave me an encouraging pat on the leg.

Mum simply said, 'Yes, I see.'

I stayed quiet.

Maybe detecting the change in the overall mood in the room, Dr Franklin suddenly changed the subject by asking my parents why they had never been to visit me in rehab during the day.

Mum was surprised. 'Jenny's husband Brad said we could only come in the evening.'

'That's not right,' Dr Franklin said. 'You can visit any time you like.'

My parents looked confused. As politely as possible, we said our goodbyes and walked outside. We were going to go to a nearby café for lunch.

As we walked, Dad turned to me and said, 'You're an intelligent girl, Jenny. They don't know how determined you are.'

Mum agreed with him.

I was blessed to have my parents. I loved them very much.

At the café, they told me they would now have to leave for Sydney. I was sad but realistic.

Mum ordered me a hamburger.

As I was eating, Dad pointed out that I had picked it up with two hands, not just one. That's how far I had come!

Three days later, I was waiting for Brad. I was finally getting out. I'd just finished saying all of my farewells and was sitting talking with some other patients in the dining room when he walked in. I only had eyes for him! He helped me check out and carried my bags for me. I was out!

We didn't go straight home, as Brad had a worm farm he wanted to deliver to Murwillumbah. I didn't mind. I was just excited to finally be free. And Brad was being nice to me, so I really didn't care where we went or what we did. That night, when we arrived home, Brad prepared us a lovely meal. Afterwards, we made love. I was glad to finally be home with my husband and relieved that he seemed happy. I felt that we would be able to save our marriage. We had a lot to celebrate.

PART 3

OUT OF REHAB

From Moodiness to Magic

When I got out, Brad wanted to throw me a big party. He was determined to make it an extravaganza. I was happy he was being so positive about my release from rehab, but when he took me shopping he began to bully me. In the produce section at the supermarket, I was trying to separate the little plastic bags that you can put your fruit into, but Brad thought I wasn't doing it fast enough. I tried not to get upset. Then I thought I would get two capsicums. Brad snapped at me, 'That won't be enough.'

I decided to get onions now and I wasn't getting them quickly enough so Brad took over. I ran out of the supermarket in tears. Wandering around aimlessly, I saw a couple of people I knew. I avoided them because I was so upset and couldn't yet speak well enough to explain what was wrong. I simply sat and waited for Brad. I was thinking that if he's like this now, just after I've come out of rehab, how would I be able to put up with him for the rest of my life? I was highly stressed. Eventually Brad came out of the supermarket and he seemed sorry.

My friend Denise had promised she would drive down from the Gold Coast to help me get the party ready and this promise kept me going. I was relieved Denise would be coming. The party was a big deal and I wanted to do it right. We had invited around sixty people, and there was a lot to do. I actually wasn't keen on having such a big party but Brad thought it was a good idea and I didn't want to disappoint him. Bill was coming up from Sydney, and I also didn't want to let him down.

On a few occasions, I had listened to a musician called Bruce Worrall. Bruce is a highly accomplished musician – he was a founding member of the Australian pop band Sherbert, had played in major musical productions such as *Jesus Christ Superstar*, *Hair* and *The Rocky Horror Picture Show*, and had also toured with the likes of the Bullamakanka Bushgrass Band and Slim Dusty. Anyway, the people of Lismore are fortunate because Bruce often plays guitar at the Lismore Car Boot Market.

I thought Bruce would be perfect for the party, so the next time the markets were on I went straight to where he was playing. As I listened from a few metres away, Bruce was reaching the end of the jazz standard *Bye Bye Blackbird*. He was performing instrumentally with the melody clearly heard against a backing arrangement – in the manner of a piano piece! – and perhaps because the melody was so beautiful many of the shoppers were singing along. 'Pack up all my care and woe, here I go, singing low, bye bye blackbird. Where somebody waits for me, sugar's sweet, so is she. Bye bye, blackbird.'

The rhythm was catchy. All the people milling around were tapping their feet and smiling.

'No one here can love and understand me,' everyone sang as Bruce played. 'Oh, what hard luck stories they all hand me. Make my bed and light the light. I'll arrive late tonight. Blackbird, bye bye.'

Bruce finished the song, and then over all the clapping and cheering he announced that he was going to take a short break.

In for a penny, in for a pound, I told myself as I worked up the courage to approach him.

'Hi. I'm Jenny,' I said. 'I like your playing.'

Bruce thanked me and smiled. He looked like a really kind man. I took a deep breath.

'Stroke,' I said next. 'Will you play at my party? I can pay you.'

Bruce looked a bit taken aback. 'Yes, I'd love to play at your party,' he said. 'But I'll do it for free.'

So that was how I got Bruce Worrall along!

And then I asked my jazz singer friend Sally Gwynne if she would sing at the party, and she said yes too. The party was going to be awesome.

Meanwhile, back at home, Brad and I had an argument about the vacuum cleaner. I can't remember the context, but it made me feel horrible. While he was outside putting up a tarpaulin, I cleaned the bathrooms. Then Brad brought some lettuces inside. He didn't think I'd be able to pull them apart and wash them. It was hard, but I managed it. I also managed to cut some tomatoes. It was a sense of achievement.

I started wondering where Denise was. It was now 5pm and I was getting worried about her. Brad and I were working frantically to get the party ready. Finally, Denise turned up; this was just as Brad was heading out to collect Bill from the airport and also while Bruce Worrall was arriving. Everything was happening at once. I showed Bruce where he could set up. Then my friend Sally walked in the door, so I introduced her to Bruce and left them to it.

Some of the rehab staff began arriving. After greeting Rose, Narelle and Helen, I took them down to the back fence and showed them our three alpacas. We fed the alpacas some hay. There was a big white male called Snowy. There was also Snowy's mother, whose name was Mumma. But my favourite was a small brown alpaca called Poppy; she was full of curiosity and seemed very interested in meeting everyone.

Just as the final wave of guests rolled in, I heard the rumble of thunder in the distance and felt a few drops of rain. It was time to put up some marquees. A number of people we knew from the local Lions Club did this, and I was grateful. Only minutes later, the skies opened up and everyone was able to take shelter. Meanwhile, several guests had ushered me out of the kitchen and were finishing the final preparations with the food. My heart filled with even more gratitude.

The party began. Bruce Worrall played tirelessly and Sally sang beautifully. Then everyone started encouraging me to sing. I was hesitant, not confident that my voice would sound all right compared to Sally's. But Sally urged me to sing. 'Come on, Jenny. You can do it!'

Taking the microphone from Sally, I stood next to Bruce and took a deep breath. Everyone was here to support me. It didn't matter if I stuffed up. I gave myself a shake. This would be all right. I sang *It Had to Be You*. I sang it for Brad. I'd performed this song many times but on this night the lyrics seemed particularly fitting.

'Some others I've seen might never be mean, might never be cross, or try to be boss, but they wouldn't do. For nobody else gave me a thrill. With all your faults, I love you still. It had to be you, wonderful you, it had to be you.'

Brad seemed to appreciate my performance. After I'd finished, he gave me a kiss. He was being so lovely now. I decided that maybe he'd only been nasty to me at the supermarket because he was feeling stressed in the lead-up to the party.

Now there was nothing to worry about. The party was a success! It was lovely and magical, and it had included all my favourite friends and relatives. I'd made up with Brad, and Denise and Bill were here to spend the night. After everyone left, the four of us sat around outside wrapped up in blankets. The rain had passed and all the stars were twinkling. I felt good vibes coming my way.

Community Rehab

After the party, it was time to get serious about my recovery. The next step in this process involved going to the Carroll Centre, a rehab service in the grounds of Lismore's St Vincent's Private Hospital.

When it was time to go for my first session, Brad took

me just down the road from our farm to a pick-up point on the Bruxner Highway. We pulled off the road and waited, and after only a couple of minutes I saw a minibus approaching. Brad helped me out of our truck just as it pulled up behind us. Two men got out and introduced themselves. They then helped me into the bus and introduced me to everyone on board. All the passengers seemed to be elderly people who had had strokes.

We then had to go and pick up several others, mainly old people. When we arrived at the Carroll Centre, it took a long time to get everyone off the bus. There were so many walking frames and wheelchairs.

It was hard being only in my forties. I felt like I was in the Twilight Zone. But I tried to be optimistic. Going to community rehab would help me improve.

Once inside the building, I checked in with the receptionist, a woman named Edith. She had cropped and dyed-red hair and looked to be in her mid-sixties. She was stern and my first impression was that she was quite the authoritarian.

'Can I get you to sign here?' she said in a way that sounded more like an order than a suggestion.

To my surprise, the first person I got to work with at the Carroll Centre was a physiotherapist named Chris, who I'd met at Ballina Rehab. I thought Chris was a good physio and he worked me hard in the pool. Afterwards I went off to have a shower. After that, I had morning tea, and then some physiotherapy, and then I was invited to play various games like quoits and darts. I was incredibly tired by the time I arrived home late that afternoon, but I felt that going to community-based rehab would be good for me.

For the next few months, I went to the Carroll Centre twice a week. Initially, I was doing a lot of hydrotherapy with Chris, which I loved. Even though he was working me hard, I was really enjoying our sessions. As I mentioned earlier, I was always happy to be in the water.

But Chris was only filling in for another person, and one day I arrived at the Carroll Centre to learn that until that permanent person arrived, I would be working with a second temporary physiotherapist who was filling in for Chris. Fortunately, this was okay by me, as this second person was a lovely German woman named Ivana who decided it was time for me to venture outside.

'Come on, Jenny,' she said in her heavy accent. 'Let's get you out on the street.'

Ivana gave me stick-like things for my hands. I wondered what they were for, and it turned out they were to help me with my gait. Apparently I had to get better at swinging my arms. To practice this, it was helpful for me to walk with an exaggerated swinging. This was difficult but I managed and it was good. While Ivana and I were walking, I also practiced my conversational skills. I wanted to know if she liked Australia, so I asked her about her life.

'I love it here,' she explained 'and I'm having an Australian boyfriend!'

I gave Ivana a huge grin. I was pleased for her, of course, but also happy that I was finally starting to have more normal conversations!

Eventually, the permanent physiotherapist arrived. Her name was Laurel. She was young and I found her quite austere and bossy. Her manner was purely professional, and I mainly recollect playing chess with her.

Mostly, I looked forward to going to the Carroll Centre so I could practice my swimming. The hydrotherapy was going well and I was feeling stronger every week. But one day Laurel said, 'You've reached your target with swimming. It's time for you to do other things.'

I was adamant that I hadn't had enough time in the pool and argued with her, but she couldn't see my point of view. She had me in the kitchen making scones and I'd had enough of that so I kicked up a stink. I flatly refused to keep making the scones. I realised I could simply go to Edith and sign out.

Edith asked me all kinds of questions but I finally got out. I phoned Brad and he came to pick me up. All up, I'd had nearly four months of community rehabilitation.

Back in the Pool

Once I'd finished with the Carroll Centre, my days became unfocused and I felt a bit lost. I was feeling particularly low one day when I received a call from the North Coast Brain Injury Rehabilitation Service, a Lismore-based organisation that operated under that name from 2007 until 2012. The friendly person on the other end of the line introduced herself and asked if she could come and see me. This person turned out to be a community rehabilitation worker called Karen Thompson, and when she arrived on my front doorstep the next day I liked her instantly.

Karen and I had morning tea and got to know one another.

As soon as Karen heard I loved swimming, she suggested we could go to water aerobics together. I was excited. A couple of days later she came to collect me, and I had my pink tracksuit on, ready to go. Karen took me to the Goonellabah Sports and Aquatic Centre, where there's a twenty-five-metre indoor heated pool. We jumped in and I couldn't stop smiling. I was so happy to be back in the water! While waiting for the class to start I tried to do laps. I felt a bit disappointed that I wasn't able to do freestyle but then told myself that Rome wasn't built in a day.

The instructor introduced herself. 'Hi, I'm Kat and we'll begin by moving around the pool.'

Everyone started walking clockwise around the pool, and then we changed direction. Kat was barking out orders. We had to run on the spot. Then it was full on.

Karen tried to get me to use my right arm. 'You have to try using it, Jenny,' she said. 'That's the only way it will become stronger.'

Next, we were supposed to be strengthening our arms by pulling ourselves up and down at the edge of the pool, and my right arm wasn't cooperating. I couldn't do it. Kat showed me how to just go halfway, and I could do that. By the time we reached the 'cool down', I was very tired but satisfied.

After that first day, I went to the pool a lot with Karen. Being at the pool was always very social, and Karen would help me make new friends. If I was in the shower room, for example, a conversation would go a bit like the following.

'Hi,' I would say to another swimmer who had smiled at me. 'I'm Jenny.'

'I'm Michelle,' the other woman would say. She would then start telling me she had three children and a husband, or whatever, before saying, 'What about you?'

And I wouldn't know what to say, so I would just say, 'Stroke!' and appeal to Karen.

Karen handled everything beautifully. 'Yes, Jenny had a stroke and can't talk well, but she's trying.'

Then Michelle or any other person I was talking to would take this in her stride. I was accepted and it made me feel normal.

Rainforest Art

Karen also took me to a place where we could do art. It was Willowbank Studio at Alstonville, on a property owned by printmaker Scott Trevelyan. Scott survived a traumatic brain injury after crashing a motorbike, and he presents art therapy sessions every fortnight. I went to quite a number of them.

On workshop days, Karen would pick me up from my place and drive me along some winding country roads before turning into a long gravel driveway. This was the entrance to the beautiful rainforest property, and the trees there reminded me of my grandparents' place. When I was little, I had loved reading books while sitting on a branch of one of the enormous trees in their back garden. Familiarity!

That first day, Karen parked in a shady spot several metres from the studio and we got out of the car. Straight away, I could smell the faint musky fragrance of the trees. There were so many of all shapes and sizes, but I'm not a botanist so I had no idea what most of them were. My brother Mark would have been able to tell me. Anyway, the place was very pleasing to the eye.

There were lots of activities at Willowbank Studio. When I first met Scott, he shook my hand and said, 'Pleased to meet you. We can do anything you want. I'm doing some printmaking at the moment. Would you like to have a go?'

I nodded. There was a brown kelpie running around and I patted her. I then got into printing.

I remember being amazed at the other people doing the art therapy. There was a truck driver who had been in a horrible accident in his truck. His brain injury was so bad that he couldn't go to the toilet on his own. I began counting my blessings! I also met a woman around my age; she had her left hand in a sling and wanted to be a wedding planner, but was having trouble thinking. I felt really sorry for her. There were several people in wheelchairs and just as many carers to help them out.

After doing some art we had a barbecue. It was a social time and it was good to hear other people's stories. There was a real feeling of camaraderie, and everyone was laughing at the kelpie, who was now running around asking for sausages and scraps.

I said, 'I had the stroke six months ago.'

A skinny blond guy yelled out, 'Try fifteen years and counting! You had your stroke only six months ago … wait and see how much you'll improve. You'll improve out of sight, Jenny!'

I remember thinking, 'This is my reality now. I am going to accept this and be the best I can be.'

More than Words

My speech started to improve – not dramatically, but I was gradually getting better at putting two or three words together. I still struggled with reading. While I could recognise individual words, I couldn't make much sense of them when they were strung together in a sentence. My Aunty Meredith gave me books by Georgette Heyer, a writer of historical romance and detective fiction. Aunty Meredith knew I adored Georgette Heyer – and because I enjoyed the material, I very slowly began to make sense of what I was reading. Eventually, I began to understand more complex novels.

A speech pathologist was coming to the house to see me. Her name was Carmel and she made me do lots of writing on endless worksheets. At one point, I went away for a holiday to Caloundra on the Sunshine Coast and Carmel asked me to keep a diary so I could practice writing while I was away. We also did role-play exercises to give me more confidence in using what she called 'conversational gambits'. These could be as simple as, 'Hi, I'm Jenny' or 'I'd like to book an appointment for Friday.' If I practiced enough, I could use these phrases with friends, family and strangers.

After I'd been working with Carmel for a couple of months, Karen noticed that my speech was improving. She took me to see a case worker called Natalie, who arranged for me to volunteer some time reading to children at the Alstonville Public Library. Natalie had explained to the library staff that I was a former high school teacher who had had a stroke.

When I first arrived at the library, one of the librarians

said she already had someone organised to read to the children but that she'd give me a go to see how I went. She introduced me to the person who was supposed to be reading and the person looked put out. I hoped she would eventually like me.

Anyway, I read to the children and it was amazing. There was no hesitation in my delivery and that was heartening. I surely could get better and better!

One of the next times I went to the library I chose to read *The Very Hungry Caterpillar* by Eric Carle.

'In the light of the moon a little egg lay on a leaf,' I read. 'One Sunday morning the warm sun came up and pop! Out of the egg came a tiny and very hungry caterpillar. He started to look for some food … '

I was sitting on a chair with a semi-circle of children in front of me. They were all sitting on the floor on a mat.

'On Monday he ate through one apple. But he was still hungry,' I continued.

As I read, out of the corner of my eye I noticed a woman strapped into a wheelchair. As soon as I had finished reading, I went over to meet her.

'Hi,' I said, and she just looked at me.

The woman's sister came over and explained that the woman couldn't talk. Her disabilities were worse than mine. I wondered what had happened to her. I was so lucky to be talking.

Being at the library was a social time and I loved it, but I went away to Sydney for a fortnight and when I returned someone higher up in the library system called to say they no longer needed me at the Alstonville Public Library. I was sad about missing out on reading to the children, partly because I felt my reading was getting better, but also because I'd always wanted children of my own. I tried to be philosophical about my disappointment. At least I'd had some happy times there.

Singing with Sally

Before my stroke, I had joined the Lismore Jazz Club. At that time, the club's president Syd Sycamore had told me about Sally – yes, the same Sally who had ended up singing at my welcome home party. But back before my stroke, I hadn't met Sally in person. I had only spoken with her over the phone. Syd had given me her number and I had called to invite her to sing with me … but before we'd had a chance to do that, I'd had the stroke.

Sally has a clear memory of that first pre-stroke conversation, and would later write that I had sounded like a 'strong, determined woman who knew what she wanted and what she was doing'. As she recalled, 'Jenny had rung me regarding starting a local group as we were both singers. Jenny sounded so dynamic and full of energy that I wasn't sure I would be able to keep up with her.'

But when Sally met me after the stroke, she observed that I was like a totally different person. 'Jenny could not speak at all and I could feel her tremendous struggle to articulate every word,' she wrote. 'But what I do remember was that she would not give up. That she would do whatever it took to get better.'

From the moment I met Sally in person I felt her full support. Warren Cleverly, a mutual friend of ours, was a guitarist, and Sally suggested that the three of us get together at her place every week for music sessions. When I asked Sally what she remembered from that time, she said that she had noticed I had a lot of difficulty singing but that I never gave up and never stopped smiling. I'm not surprised that I was smiling so much at those sessions; I really did feel that music was making me well.

Taking Flight

I was excited! My brother John and his wife Kirsty were coming to see me. They were coming all the way from Darwin with their two children: four-year-old Jack and two-year-old Riley. I hadn't seen the children since before I'd had my stroke. I was pacing up and down in our house at Alstonvale. I couldn't wait for them to arrive.

When they finally arrived, I hugged them all. It should have been a good time, but Brad was determined to be cross with everyone. We all tried to take Brad's bad mood in our stride. That night, Kirsty was in the kitchen making a roast for us. I was trying to help her but was having trouble with my right arm. Brad suddenly appeared and said, 'Use your fucking arm.'

Kirsty was shocked. 'You can tell her gently,' she said.

John walked away. Perhaps he was just trying to keep calm and mind his own business.

After dinner, the children ran outside. We were all sitting on the patio watching them play. I had given them some saucepans to use as toys. It was hilarious. The children were putting the saucepans on their heads! Brad laughed at that, and everything seemed fine. Kirsty and John were making a big effort to be kind to Brad. It was all going smoothly, finally.

But later that night, not long after the children went to bed, I heard a loud argument coming from the kitchen. I went to find out why everyone was shouting and heard something about putting my father into a nursing home. Apparently Brad wanted this to happen. I was distraught. Everyone was so upset. There was no resolution to the argument. In the end, Brad said he wanted my brother and his family to leave. Even though John and Kirsty had been intending to stay for a few days, they said they would leave the next morning.

I remember lying in bed that night, wide awake. Brad was in a deep sleep, with his arm flung across my body like a dead weight. I had lost all respect for him. If he was going to be like this with my family, everyone would be too uncomfortable to come and visit me.

The next day Brad made himself scarce. I'd arranged to meet friends at a French restaurant, so I called them to check if my brother and his family could come, too. My friends said yes. We were all planning to leave my house at the same time but Kirsty discovered Jack had drawn on the leather lounge with a texta, and she was determined to clean it off. By the time the lounge was back in good condition, the lunch was almost over. John, Kirsty and the kids still dropped in at the restaurant, though, to say goodbye. I was sorry to see them go. I hugged them tightly, especially my brother. Later, I learnt that a couple of hours after we had said goodbye, Kirsty had rung my good friend Jane to ask her to keep an eye on me.

When I was talking to Jane on the phone the next day, I couldn't stop crying. Jane worked as a travel agent. Through my sobs, she could make out that I was saying, 'Leave … him.'

Jane knew how serious my marital problems were, and having talked to Kirsty, she felt it was time to act. Jane booked me a flight to Sydney. She then drove from her home in Ballina, picked me up from Alstonvale, and took me to Ballina airport. She put me on a plane.

But when I was staying in Sydney with my parents, Brad's friend Bill came over to see me. I told him that I was leaving Brad, but Bill persuaded me to give Brad another chance. Next thing I knew, Brad was on the phone, saying how shocked he was that I was planning on leaving him. I felt sorry for him. I could hear so much grief in his voice and began thinking of how lonely he would be on the farm by himself. Sadly, our beautiful dog Millie had been hit by a car and killed a few months earlier, so he no longer even had Millie for company. Even though Brad had bought Millie for me, he had formed a deep bond with her and was grief stricken when she died.

I suddenly missed him. Perhaps I was giving up too easily? I thought I would have another attempt at making it work.

A few days later, when I flew back into Ballina, I was feeling nervous. I wondered how Brad would react. I crossed the tarmac in trepidation, walked through the doors of the airport hangar and looked around. Brad came over to me, and he looked nervous too. He gave me a kiss. As we waited by the luggage carousel for my bag, he told me he had booked us a table for lunch at the pub in Eltham. It was a lovely country pub and a favourite of mine. At the pub, we got on well and we were laughing. When we got home we made love.

Yes, We Have No Bananas

Not long after my reconciliation with Brad, I started rehearsing with the Lismore Symphony Orchestra. Every two years, the orchestra staged a production of Handel's *Messiah*, and the director wanted singers for that year's performances. I was keen to volunteer. After all, even though I couldn't speak fluently, I could sing! The music was powerful and stirring. I went to rehearsals and was given the top soprano part, and I could sing it. I felt free of all cares and worries while I was singing.

Meanwhile, any time I was at home, I was still being extremely careful about everything I did and said. I did not want to upset Brad, but I wasn't always successful. One night I was cooking a curry when I realised we didn't have any bananas. Whenever I make curry, I like to sprinkle flakes of coconut and slices of banana on top, as a garnish. It was getting dark but I didn't want to ask Brad for help because I knew he'd have a go at me.

I decided to walk the 200 metres or so down our road to the nearest fruit stall. Relief! There were two bananas left. I dropped a dollar coin into the honesty box attached to the side of the stall.

In retrospect, I can see how pathetic it was to be filled with trepidation because we'd run out of bananas. How crazy that I felt I couldn't communicate something so basic without fear of making Brad angry. I began being honest with myself;

there was something seriously wrong with our relationship.

Around this time, I bought Brad a ticket to the *Messiah* production. I hoped he would come along to see me doing something I loved. After all, I remember how much he had enjoyed watching me perform with choirs in Sydney before we were married. But when the day came, Brad said he wanted to work instead. I felt that he resented me going out, but I was determined to help make the production a success. I decided that I would put my troubles aside and sing my heart out.

So I rang up Jane and offered her Brad's ticket. She was worried about me and accepted at once. That night, my friend Helen picked me up. I told her I was really sad that Brad wouldn't come. I was singing in a beautiful production and this was a big deal to me.

The *Messiah* was at Lismore City Hall. At interval, as soon as I saw Jane I burst into tears. She led me to a quiet corner and said, 'You can't go on like this, Jenny. If it isn't working, there's no crime in calling it quits.'

I had had enough. I was going to leave him. I went on with singing the *Messiah* and my heart was breaking. Afterwards, all my friends were telling me, 'Well done!' and making a fuss over me. I couldn't say I was going to leave Brad. I was terrified.

Helen and her husband drove me home. On the way, I picked up some Chinese takeaway. When I walked in the door, I said to Brad, 'Hi! I got takeout!'

I heard a terse reply. 'I don't want any. I already have my dinner here.'

He was stirring something in a saucepan. Apparently he

was making his own dinner.

So I fetched a plate and I ate my takeout. I was exhausted. Brad didn't ask me how I went in the performance. That night, I slept far away from him in our bed.

Going Somewhere?

I wasn't getting well. I knew that to get well I had to leave Brad. I finally conceded I was in a toxic relationship. I had to get out.

The next morning when Brad was busy outside, I started packing. But he came into our bedroom right when I was in the middle of sorting out my clothes and snapped, 'What are you doing?'

I stayed calm. 'I'm leaving you.'

'Oh, right,' he said. 'Not this again.' He proceeded to unpack my cases.

I kept folding clothes. He kept unpacking my cases.

Eventually, I sat on the bed, not knowing what to do.

Brad said, 'You really are selfish. Don't go anywhere until we sort this out.'

I thought he was selfish for not coming to hear me sing. I saw him for who he was: a little man afraid of his own shadow.

'I have to go out,' he said. 'Don't do anything until I get back.'

And that was the last time I saw Brad.

Because I continued to pack. And as soon as I heard his car drive out onto the road, I rang Jane to tell her she had to arrange a flight for me. But Jane couldn't come straight away so I rang my friend Sally, and she booked me a flight and came over.

It was such a relief when she finally arrived.

I had four big bags because I wasn't planning to return. Sally was putting them in the boot of her car when a courier turned up at our house with some packages for Brad.

'Going somewhere?' he asked.

'Sydney,' I said, and I got in the car with Sally.

PART 4

Free to Fly

Debriefing

I didn't know what I was going to do. I had left Brad. I don't think he ever believed I would actually go, but I had suffered enough verbal abuse to understand I wouldn't get well while living with his constant mood swings. With Brad, I would never know what I was going to get: a cheery Brad or an angry Brad. I had lost the dream of 'happily ever after'. It had only been a pipe dream.

Of course, this is only my perspective and it is probably different to Brad's. But what has helped me have confidence in my decision is the positive reinforcement I've received from family, friends and health care professionals. Jane, for example, told me several times in the months following my stroke that she was concerned about Brad's inability to look after me and support me in my time of need, saying that Brad 'always seemed to be complaining about taking you to rehab and doing anything for you, as though this tragedy that had happened to you was something that had really happened to him'.

Jane felt so strongly about this opinion that she gave me permission to quote her in this book. 'This was a huge thing for anyone to go through,' she said, 'let alone at your young age, and with the lack of support you experienced from the person who was supposed to be your greatest ally. It was a hard time, I know.'

It was indeed a hard time, there's no doubt about that, but I don't wish Brad any ill will. In his own way he had tried to help me, I guess, especially during my second and third months in rehab. This is when he had brought me home each weekend and had insisted on giving me the electrical muscle stimulation when the physiotherapists weren't around to assist me – even when I argued that I couldn't be bothered. And yes, we had been happy together initially. I had loved him. But in the end, we just weren't compatible, and I valued myself more.

Learning Curve

So there I was, living back in Sydney with my parents. Even though I felt a sense of relief now that I could get well, I still felt broken-hearted, and I didn't have any idea about what I was going to do.

My parents wanted to help. Mum took me to St George Public Hospital to see the renowned rehabilitation specialist Dr Andrew Cole, who was a friend of Dad's. Dr Cole was a tall grey-haired man who was very nice to me. My brother John was there, too. I felt I was in safe hands. Dr Cole gave me a thorough examination and I managed to make myself understood. Dr Cole explained that even though I had what he called 'severe expressive dysphasia', he knew I understood everything that was being said to me. I felt so lucky! How easily I could've ended up stuck in a wheelchair with no comprehension of anything going on around me. Dr Cole said he would refer me to excellent speech and occupational therapists. I nodded. I had the rest of my life to live. I wanted to get well.

A week or so later I had an appointment with a speech therapist at St George Hospital in Kogarah. Her name was Claire Piggot and she was an excellent speech therapist; I could see why Dr Cole had recommended her. Afterwards, I was having a coffee at a nearby café, and was wondering what to do with my life. I felt lost. How would I earn a living? I started feeling depressed … then I thought, 'Damn it, I'll wander over to St George TAFE.'

The TAFE building was only a five-minute walk away. I found the office. There were all sorts of brochures there and I flicked through them. I wasn't paying much attention to the brochures until I saw one describing a Certificate IV in Community Services that focussed on Lifestyle and Leisure. I got excited!

The brochure explained that the course taught participants how to plan activities for clients in the community services, health and aged care sectors. One of the jobs I could apply for if I completed the course was the role of an activities officer in an aged care facility. This really interested me! I liked elderly people and I thought that with my teaching experience that type of job would really suit me.

It was busy in the office and there were students everywhere. I lined up. When I reached the reception desk I managed to tell them that I wanted to see someone about a course and that I had had a stroke. Straight away, they got hold of a Disability Liaison Officer, who introduced herself as Kate Gillian and ushered me into her office. Once Kate and I were sitting looking at each other across her desk, she asked me how she could help.

I handed her the brochure. 'Want to do this,' I said slowly. I then somehow managed to explain that I'd had a stroke in the previous year.

Kate was wonderful. She could sense how much I wanted to do the course. Before I knew it, I was enrolled – with the fees fully covered because Kate told me I was eligible for a government subsidy. I was amazed at how fast everything was happening. I felt like I was getting somewhere. I was so happy.

On my way home I kept thinking about how much I wanted to be an activities officer in aged care. I had met so many wise older people in rehab. I liked their company. They had helped me get through some very rough times.

Two weeks later I started at TAFE. I had a note taker. Her name was Marie and she had red hair. We sat next to each other in the classroom and had just started chatting when the acting head teacher walked in. Her name was Margaret Murphy, and years later she would confess that initially, although she could see I was very determined, she had had some reservations about my ability to complete the course.

Anyway, I was determined to give it my best shot. Going to TAFE was challenging but I was happy to be out in the world again, and it was good to have something to concentrate on. I was studying with a diverse range of students; some were just out of school but others were a lot older. One older student was Diane Hollis. She was energetic and friendly. We became friends.

Giving Back

Diane ended up getting a job at a small aged care facility called Bethlehem House. It was in Kogarah and she loved it. I asked Diane if she thought I could do my TAFE work placement there and she said yes, so we organised it.

The old people were lovely. There was one man in particular who caught my attention. His name was John. He was a big man and had sandy hair. He was in his mid-sixties and had had a stroke. Although John didn't have any speech difficulties, he couldn't use his left arm at all and was having trouble looking after himself. I did my case study on him.

There were other people, too. In interacting with them I managed to make myself understood. We sang together. One client liked country music. He was a big blonde man and was nice to me. He was lovely and always eager to chat. I actually suspected that he used to lie in wait for me. He was lonely and his children didn't visit him much. I resolved to put on a Country Music Day. It was a lot of work but the brightness on his face was worth it. I was really enjoying my placement at Bethlehem House and the clients there were friends to me. Some were as sharp as tacks but others were living with dementia, and no one seemed to mind if I couldn't think of a word and had to start over again. They got me out of myself.

Some friends at TAFE had had a lot of success singing with dementia-care clients. One day in class they did a presentation about their methods using music. After I told them I wanted to do what they were doing, they kindly burnt me a copy of a Toni Lamond sing-along CD they always used. I was excited. Every Friday after my TAFE classes were over, I'd go straight to Bethlehem House and play the CD so the clients and I could sing together. The joy on everyone's faces was priceless. We'd sing all the old songs from the war years, like *White Cliffs of Dover* and *We'll Meet Again*.

Besides singing, I also did other activities at Bethlehem House and also at another respite centre where I volunteered for about eighteen months. This second place was at Calgary Health Care in Kogarah, and is now called Mary Potter House – although it had a different name back then. At both places, I gave hand massages, played games of 'hangman' on a whiteboard, and also called the numbers for bingo. Running the games of hangman and calling the bingo required a lot of talking, so these activities were the hardest ones to do. I really had to concentrate!

Although I was volunteering at two respite centres, my formal work placement was at Bethlehem House. I was simply doing the additional volunteering because I loved the work so much. By helping out the elderly people, I was contributing to the wider community – and I was happy to feel useful. As Gandhi[1] once said, 'The best way to find yourself is to lose yourself in the service of others.' I really enjoyed the feeling of 'giving back'.

But when it came to preparing my final report about

that work placement, I found it incredibly difficult to put my thoughts in order. Fortunately, my wonderful study buddy, Diane, was there to help me.

'Shove over and I'll do the writing for you,' she said. Diane was a good friend. She helped me get my assignments done, and I ended up passing the course with a credit.

Teaching Again?

The acting head teacher, Margaret Murphy, told me she was impressed that I had pushed through my impatience and frustration to do what needed to be done to complete the certificate.

'Many people in your situation don't finish the course,' she told me. 'I was amazed that you found ways to adjust to the demands of studying and followed through with your efforts.'

But what could I do now that I had finished studying? Sitting across the desk from Margaret in her office, we discussed possible plans for my future. Haltingly, I managed to explain to her that I still really wanted to teach again but didn't know if I could do it.

'Hmm,' she said, thinking hard. 'Perhaps you could do a certificate course in Individual Support (Disability), as it includes a component for teaching.' She got out a brochure and handed it to me.

'Yes, I want to teach again,' I said. 'But I have a problem getting my speech out.'

Margaret understood. 'Yes, I'm aware of that – but nothing ventured, nothing gained.' She thought for another moment and then told me about Cairnsfoot School, which was based in Arncliffe at that time and catered for children with moderate to severe intellectual disabilities. 'I'll give them a call for you,' she promised.

The very next week, I went along to the school to introduce myself to a teacher called Wendy Brown, and she suggested that I come back the following term to begin my work placement, which is exactly what I did.

Even though Cairnsfoot School was different to any other school I'd known, it was great to get back into an educational environment. On my first full day there, I arrived at 7.30 am. I was so excited! After checking in at the front office I went to find Wendy.

When I found her, she was at the front of the school and was busy helping students out of minibuses. Some of the pupils were only in kindergarten. Others were in Year 12.

'Hi, Jenny!' Wendy said. 'I'll be right with you.'

Wendy knew my placement was for three weeks, and she wanted to give me experience with children of all ages and abilities during that relatively short time. She started me off in a class for children who were all about eight years old. There were only seven students and they were all boys, and the atmosphere was chaotic. First, I helped the kids put their lunch boxes in a fridge, and all of them were clamouring for my attention. Happy to be caught up in the excitement, I took my cues from Wendy, who seemed to have a beautiful rapport with every student. Next, we gave the boys worksheets that they could colour in. I was enjoying all the energy in the room. I began thinking I could really do this.

One little boy completed his worksheet. Crouching down beside him, I told him I liked the colours he had used. I stuck a shiny little gold star on his work … and he bit me! I didn't know what to do. Even now, I can't remember what I did. I had felt so shocked. But I told myself that things were bound to improve. After all, I'd be doing Drama with the boys the next day, and that was my specialty.

I'd actually taught Drama with a group of special needs students back when I was working at Lismore High School, so I felt quite confident. I only needed to teach for half an hour, and figured that with all my experience of more than twenty years I could teach Drama off the top of my head.

The next morning, Wendy told the children, 'Now, Miss Sheldon is going to take you for Drama.'

I was excited and hopeful. *If I can do this, I'll be able to work as a Drama teacher for students with special needs*, I thought.

I took over. I said, 'Squat down.' I demonstrated. 'We will be little trees, and we will grow into big trees!' For about two minutes, everyone was busy being trees. The room was calm.

But then my aphasia came to bite me. One child started running around the room and then a couple of others followed. Within moments, every child was running around. Chaos had erupted, and I couldn't think of anything to say. It was such a highly stressful situation and I couldn't speak. Disaster!

Wendy asked me if she could take over.

I nodded, feeling very upset.

The next day, I thought I would have more luck working with a largely non-verbal class of kindergarten students. As these students couldn't feed themselves, I helped feed them their fruit, which included bananas, kiwi fruit, apples and pears, and which they were meant to try, and to ask for. I also supervised them on the playground equipment. One little boy had developed an attachment to me and he wanted to sit on my knee. I obliged and we sat there for a long time.

Over the next three weeks I attended a number of other classes, including a class for young teenagers who were all on the autism spectrum. I remember one particular thirteen-year-old girl who was blonde with blue eyes. The moment the teacher's back was turned she ran away. One of the disability support officers went after her. The officer was big and strong, and I realised that was good, as she needed to restrain the student. I began to question if I was the right person for this kind of job.

The last straw came on the final Friday. Droves of people were going home and the front of the school was crowded. A large older boy came out of nowhere and suddenly had me in a headlock. I began to choke. A teacher quickly came to my defence. If he hadn't, I hate to think what would have happened. I decided then and there not to teach again.

Meeting Marina

It was depressing to think the disability course hadn't worked out and that I was finally giving up my dream of returning to teaching, but at least I now knew for certain I was better off working with elderly people. I thought they were much more steady. And besides, I had completed the relevant TAFE certification for working with older people, and I knew without a doubt that working with older people was much easier for me than working with kids!

I decided to tell Margaret Murphy. I went to her office and we had a good talk. She said, 'I don't know why you wanted to teach children, anyway.'

I said, 'I thought I could do Drama with special needs kids but it didn't work out.'

Margaret smiled at me from across her desk. 'Hammond-Care is looking for volunteers to work with people living with dementia. Why don't you do that?'

I nodded.

She made the phone call.

The following week, which was late in November 2009, I set out to drive to HammondCare, which was located at Hammondville, in southwestern Sydney. Although I took a few wrong turns on the way, I eventually arrived and stepped out of the car full of confidence. In the main office, a woman named Sue made me feel very welcome.

'Hi, Jenny! I've heard good things about you,' she said, smiling. 'Step into my office.'

We had a friendly chat about the facility and what kind of things I could do to help out, and before I knew it Sue was saying, 'Well, it's just about lunchtime. You can meet Marina and the residents you'll be looking after.'

And that's how I met the wonderful Marina. I walked into the dining room and was immediately accosted by an elderly lady named Thelma who seemed to think I was her daughter. I went along with it. I had just helped Thelma sit down at a table where her lunch was being served when Marina came up to introduce herself. I liked what I saw. Marina was of Italian heritage, and was blonde, blue-eyed and slim. I instantly felt that I could work with her. Over the rest of the day, I watched her with the residents; she treated them all like they were her parents.

As Marina worked, she explained that HammondCare wouldn't need me until January. I was actually relieved to hear that, as I would now be able to have a holiday. When I came back to HammondCare after my holiday, I developed a firm friendship with Marina and we ended up working together for two years – Marina in a paid position, with me in a voluntary capacity. Marina did try to get me a paid position there, but because there was heavy lifting involved it turned out I wasn't eligible.

A couple of years later, I would eventually find paid work in aged care as an activities officer. But this would be when I moved back up to the far north coast for a couple of years from 2012 and goes beyond my story here.

Driven to Drive

A week or so before I had left rehab, a neuropsychologist had told me I would never be able to drive again. Fancy telling me that! At the time I just looked at her and said nothing, but in my mind I was throwing darts at her. Although I understand she probably believed she was being realistic, she could have been a lot kinder. I couldn't imagine not driving!

I went to talk with some of the nurses, feeling crazy with

grief. They listened and sympathised. I then went to my room and tried adding up numbers to distract myself. After a while, I began telling myself over and over, 'Let's just wait and see about that!' I decided I would do everything I possibly could to get back on the road. Of course, if there was a chance I was going to be a danger to other people on the roads then I didn't want to drive. But I felt I would be okay, and I had to try.

As I mentioned earlier, in 2009 I had begun seeing Dr Andrew Cole, the rehabilitation expert in Sydney. Dr Cole felt confident that I would eventually be able to get back behind the wheel, and arranged for a neurophysiologist to come to my house to help me attempt to regain my licence.

I wish I could remember this neurophysiologist's name. He had a nice bedside manner and did a lot of tests before telling me, 'The right hand is a bit of a worry, but there are things you can do to work around it.'

The next thing I knew, the neurophysiologist was handing me a referral to the Driver Assessment and Retraining Service at Calgary Healthcare in Kogarah. As he passed me this very important piece of paper, he said, 'I'm hopeful that you'll be able to drive, Jenny. Good luck!'

At Kogarah, I began working with an occupational therapist who specialised in driving rehabilitation. This person's job was to figure out the various impacts my medical condition was having on my ability to drive safely and legally, and then to train me in a modified vehicle so I could work towards getting my licence back and regaining my independence!

Anyway, that's how I got Dean Jones. I was going to work with him for a year, and I was ecstatic!

Once I was in a training car with Dean, he wanted to see if I could brake. I was able to do that, and he was pleased. I was going along well until he asked me to make a right turn and I made a left turn instead.

Dean remained calm. 'No, Jenny,' he said gently. 'I said right, not left'.

I was aghast. 'Sorry! I'm getting mixed up. Since my stroke I don't know my right from my left.'

Dean was a kind person. 'That's okay. Perhaps just try to remember that your good hand is left and your bad hand is right.'

I tried to remember that idea, and it helped a bit. Although I still get mixed up today.

Dean realised how much trouble I was having, even with his patient help. He continued, 'That's perfectly normal, Jenny. For now, how about I simply point out which way to turn?'

We proceeded with the lesson.

After a few weeks of training, Dean told me that although he didn't think I would be able to drive with both hands, he thought that maybe I could practice steering on arcade driving games. So I did that, going into arcades as much as I could and practicing my steering.

But eventually, I had to concede that I wasn't able to drive with both hands. This wasn't the end of my quest to get my licence, though, as there didn't seem to be a problem Dean couldn't work around. He arranged for me to try driving with a device called a Spinmaster. This enabled me to use the steering wheel with one hand! And the Spinmaster was fitted with another device called a PME Easyspin, which fits onto the steering wheel of a car to allow one-handed control of indicators and other functions such as the headlight and horn. These devices were amazing. I soon got the hang of them. My left hand could do all the work, and I also had a special cushion I could rest my right arm on.

Finally, Dean told me I could go for my driving test.

But I have a confession to make. I'm scared of driving tests. When I was twenty-seven, I thought it would be easy to get my licence. I went along to the testing venue full of optimism … and then failed nine driving tests in a row.

Then, during a lesson, I was following what the driving instructor was telling me and had just pulled up at a stop sign when a taxi seemed to come out of nowhere. It collected me. My car was slammed into a spin and ended up crashing through a brick fence at the front of someone's house. I hit my head on the windscreen and had a thumping headache, so now I had to go to the hospital to get checked out. By that point, even though the accident wasn't my fault, I decided the universe was telling me I wasn't meant to get my licence. But I tried again and got it.

Now here I was, nearly a year and a half after my stroke, and about to sit a driving test again. So you can probably imagine how much trepidation I was feeling. It was October 2009. First, I had to drive at forty kilometres per hour. But I was nervous and I drove too fast. Other than that, I'd done everything right, but of course I didn't pass.

Then on my third try at getting my driving licence since my stroke, I got it.

Of course, I had to get my own Spinmaster and PME

Easyspin, which are made by a company called PME Auto Conversions at Hornsby Heights. The 'PME' stands for 'Problem Management Engineering', and a man called Bill Georgas started the business in 1989 after becoming a paraplegic. Bill had previous experience as an engineer, so when the hand controls fitted to his car failed to meet his expectations he set about creating his own devices. Before long, he began making driving aids for other people living with disabilities.

Anyway, after I passed my driving test, Mum made an appointment for us to go to PME Auto Conversions. She drove me out there in my car, and Bill and his team fitted the driving aids to the steering wheel. It was inspiring to meet Bill. He was in a wheelchair and was running a highly successful business. Bill reckons that if there's a way to work around a physical challenge, he'll find it. I liked his fighting spirit. He was making a huge difference to people's lives by getting hundreds drivers back on the road.

And guess what? I became one of those drivers! Because once Bill was finished with my car, Mum hopped into the passenger seat and I was the one who drove us all the way home!

Being back on the road boosted my confidence and made me much more independent. My horizons broadened literally and figuratively!

Having my own transport enabled me to get more involved with friends, and at that stage in my life I was especially grateful to be spending time with those friends who played a huge part in my recovery – especially because our bonds developed as we took part in creative hobbies like singing and acting.

Singing Friends

When it came to singing after my stroke, I decided to join a Cronulla-based community choir called the Sea Naturals. Well-known Sydney choir director Stuart Davis started the group, which is now directed by Lanneke Jones. Joining this choir was one of the best things I'd done since moving back to Sydney, as I made so many new friends to sing with. We sang everything from African music and jazz to pop and gospel. After rehearsals, we always had a cup of tea together.

One friend I met through the Sea Naturals was a very cheerful man named Laurie Abela. The first time I met him I couldn't wait to get to know him better. The opportunity arose when I wanted to go to the Sydney Writers Festival to see Norman Doidge, the author of *The Brain That Changes Itself*. I wanted to buy his book and hear him speak. Laurie said he would come with me. When we were arranging the outing, he revealed that he had multiple sclerosis and that he wasn't letting the condition get him down. I admired his attitude and we became firm friends.

One afternoon when I was doing voluntary work in an aged care centre, I had a seizure. Mum was away at the time so I called Laurie and he took me to a doctor and then to St George Hospital, where he sat with me in the emergency department while the staff there gave me some tests. After that day I wasn't allowed to drive for six months, so Laurie drove me to choir rehearsals through that entire period. I was so grateful. He is a very good friend.

Other firm friends who were a great help in my recovery

were Uta Mihm, and Josie and Colin Nicholson. These friends had been in the choir that had performed at my wedding but I hadn't seen them much since moving up north with Brad. But when they heard I'd had a stroke and had returned to Sydney, they came back into my life and were generous with me.

Uta encouraged me to join a social group with her, and we'd meet up at piano bars to listen to jazz. One time, I even joined Uta in Melbourne so we could attend the Melbourne Comedy Festival. Being out and about with Uta brought plenty of friendship, music and laughter into my life. Meanwhile, when I didn't feel up to driving, Josie and Colin would give me rides to choir events. Sometimes I even stayed overnight at their place. They were such lovely people I never would have met if it wasn't for singing.

Theatre Buddies

Drama also played a big part in my recovery thanks to other dear friends such as Vicki Pillinger and Bronwyn Green, whose name when we first met was Bronwyn Laney. Vicki was the daughter of my dad's secretary. She was a chef, and I became friends with her when she was sharing a house with my brother Mark. Eventually, I would go on to share two houses with her.

But in the meantime, back in 1992, it was through Vicki that I met Bronwyn, a vivacious primary school teacher with beautiful jet-black hair and green eyes. Vicki had invited Bronwyn along to my parents' house on Christmas Day, and right from the first moment I had found her hilarious and wanted to get to know her better. Anyway, luckily for me Bronwyn was happy to exchange phone numbers, because we went on to become close friends.

Bronwyn and I went away a lot together, and when Mark died in 1998 she took great care of me. She was so thoughtful. In the year 2000, more than 250,000 people came together to walk across Sydney Harbour Bridge in what was called The People's Walk for Reconciliation. The walk enabled people to show their support for the process of reconciliation between Indigenous Australians and others. It was Bronwyn's idea for us to do it together as a way of honouring my brother's memory. After all, as I mentioned earlier, Mark had dedicated his career to improving the welfare of Indigenous Australians.

Bronwyn's happiness was always important to me, so in 1998 I was delighted when she met a lovely man named Colin Green (through a former boyfriend!) … and then married him in 2003 and had their daughter Grace in the same year. But tragically, Colin died from a heart attack in 2015. I still miss him today. Like Bronwyn, Colin always made me laugh. He was forever calling me 'spastic'. I liked the way he wasn't afraid to tease me; he wouldn't let me get too serious.

Despite her own grief, Bronwyn is a compassionate listener. Actually, she has always been like that. After my stroke, I would ring her up and struggle to get some words out. Basically I would just try to say any word at all just so she would know it was me, and then she would say something like, 'Jenny, do you want me to take over? Would you like me to just talk for a while?' Then she'd always say something to crack me up.

Bronwyn loved being involved with the theatre. Once I had moved back to Sydney after leaving Brad, I found she was one of a small team of women who produced a play I could take part in. Called *Renovations*, the play was written by one of the women, Heather Pitt, who would also go on to direct it.

At the heart of the play would be four different monologues, each written by the actor who would be performing that particular speech. The monologues were about themes relating to overhauling, remodelling, and improvement – but these themes didn't relate to buildings; they were more about the challenges of repairing of one's own body, mind and soul. Everyone wanted me to do one of the monologues, and they said they would help me write it.

Aside from Bronwyn and Heather, the other fabulous women who came together to create the show were Lou Deibe, Angela Miles, Pauline Burnett, Fiona Ross and Linda Mosey. All the women knew each other from attending church on the Northern Beaches, and they decided they would stage their play at local churches, RSL clubs and schools. Best of all, they decided that they would donate all the proceeds from *Renovations* to the Stroke Foundation. I was excited about being involved!

But this workshopping of the play was happening in 2008, only a year after my stroke, and even though I was going for regular and intensive speech therapy, I was having a lot of trouble delivering my lines. At speech therapy I could re-start words if I got confused, but the idea of stammering on stage made me really anxious. So I finally said, 'I can't.' And it wasn't just my non-fluent aphasia that made me pull out. I was living in Blakehurst at the time, and all the rehearsals were being held on the Northern Beaches.

But all was not lost. The friends who were making the play decided they would all perform different aspects of my role on my behalf, while at the same time devising a way for me to still be personally involved without the need to attend rehearsals and deliver my lines under pressure. Heather Pitt announced that she would help me make a video that would be screened as part of the play! With Heather's help, I wrote the script for the video. The script was based on the concept of a stroke survivor working as a teacher, and all the funny things that could go wrong. But it also showed the things that could go right.

Bronwyn decided my monologue would hinge around a butterfly motif, as my recovery from stroke was like a metamorphosis – and not only in a physical sense, but also in terms of restoring my spirit.

During the play, as the video appeared on a big screen behind the performers, each person took a turn acting out a different episode from my life, such as the lead-up to my stroke, the stroke itself, and the challenges I was facing in my recovery. I loved how the actors conveyed the ways I had learnt to use my body and voice since the stroke, and how I was adapting to my new life.

Several months later, the play opened to packed audiences. It was then staged a few more times for full houses across the varied venues I mentioned earlier, and then there was one special performance an entire year later.

Although I went to every performance, two stand out in my memory. One was the single performance held a year later, in 2010. I took my mother, and she burst into tears at the end.

She'd been under pressure as my father had recently died, and I guess she was also sad about everything I'd gone through. The play was quite confronting for her to watch. The other memorable night was during the major run of the play in 2009, when I drove all the way to the Northern Beaches and back by myself. This felt like a big achievement, made all the more poignant by the fact that my character in the video talked about learning to drive again after her stroke.

Being involved in the play was the most wonderful experience. I was so happy that all the money went to the Stroke Foundation, and also that Colin and his daughter Grace could come along and see the play before Colin died. It's so terribly sad that Bronwyn and Grace lost this beautiful man. Col was larger than life, and he loved his wife and daughter so much.

But what's strange is that thinking back now to the final night of the play, I can suddenly remember something I had long forgotten: Bronwyn pulling me aside afterwards.

'Thank you, Bron,' I said, and hugged her.

She hugged me back. 'I bought you a present.'

I eagerly unwrapped it. Inside the tissue paper was a butterfly necklace and it was lovely, shaped exactly like a butterfly. I put it on with her help and she said, 'Now you can be free.'

With the butterfly necklace on, I felt that everything was bound to turn out all right.

Silver Linings

Late in 2013, my brother and I begged Mum to go on a European cruise with her sister Del. Mum had been through so much over the previous few years. Dad had developed dementia in the years before his death, and at the same time had also undergone several surgeries for a range of diseases from bowel cancer to prostate cancer. Mum had looked after him the entire time. We thought it would be good for her to get away, and she finally agreed.

While Mum was in Europe, I decided to go to the opening of the Archibald Prize exhibition at the Art Gallery of NSW. I would meet some friends there, and after looking at the portraits we would listen to the live jazz performance that would take place as part of the opening celebrations.

I planned to arrive at the gallery early so I'd have the opportunity to look at some other exhibitions before meeting my friends. I drove to Kogarah Station, got the train to Martin Place and then walked to the gallery from there. First, I wanted to see some Australian art. I thought it would be good to find a painting by the painter, sculptor and art teacher called Frank Hinder, as I'd inherited one of his paintings through my grandfather. Bamps had taught Botany at the University of Sydney, which is where Frank Hinder was teaching art. Frank and Bamps had been good friends, and my grandmother had bought the painting as a present for Bamps.

I had cheap boots on. I don't buy cheap boots now. Because you guessed it: the floor was slippery. I remember telling myself to be careful because I didn't want to slip. I was walking across the wooden floor looking for a Frank Hinder painting and that's when I went down with a thud, actually putting out my bad right arm to break my fall.

The gallery visitors were aghast. The security guard

rushed over and said, 'Are you all right?' I was down on the floor stunned. He helped me to get up again and walked me over to a couch. I was perplexed. If the floor was slippery, surely there should have been a warning sign.

My right arm was hurting like hell. I was in shock. I assessed my other body parts. Apart from my arm, I seemed to be okay.

The security guard looked worried. 'Are you sure you're all right?'

I said, 'Yes. I'm all right. I think I'll just have a coffee.'

Still shaking, I went down to the café. Once there, I called over a waitress and told her I needed medical attention. Help came immediately and as a first aid officer patched me up, she told me, 'You'll need to go to your doctor to see if that arm is all right.'

Great, I thought. Another visit to the doctor.

I went to see if my friends had arrived. They had. And they were appalled at what had happened. My friend Kevin got me a glass of champagne and proceeded to make me feel better. I walked around the Archibald Prize exhibition with my friends and listened to the speech from the winning artist. Then we listened to the jazz. I actually had a good time.

When I eventually got back to Kogarah, my car wouldn't start. It had a flat battery! As I waited for the NRMA, I thought, *Oh dear, this night is turning into a series of accidents.*

Once the NRMA had started my car, I found that I could drive. After all, my left arm was okay and I never used my right arm to drive anyway. Remember I had those driving aids on my steering wheel? At least that was something I had in my favour!

The next day I contacted my cousin Bruce, who's a doctor, and we arranged to meet straight away at his practice in Abbotsford. I was glad to be going there. When Bruce examined me, he said my arm would have to be x-rayed. The long and the short of it was that I had a broken arm.

I won't bother with the detail of how I had my arm fixed. But what was strange was that since having the stroke, even though I had generally felt that my right arm was largely useless, I now really missed using it!

Once the bone had healed, I went to Southern Hand Therapy in Kogarah, where a team of physiotherapists and occupational therapists gave me a series of exercises, including ones that involved picking up a plastic drinking glass and placing it upside down, and putting elastic bands on and off different items. I went to Southern Hand Therapy three times. On the final time the woman said, 'I can't do anything more for you, Jenny. Just practice.'

I was disappointed. 'Oh, isn't there anything else you can do?'

This woman knew I had had a stroke.

She thought harder. 'Hmm. There is a place called the Advance Rehab Centre but it's in St Leonards.'

I nodded. 'I can drive there. What are the details?'

And that's how I found out about the Advance Rehab Centre, which was wonderful, and which I would recommend to anybody.

Flying Colours

When the time for my first appointment arrived, Mum was back from her cruise. She came with me on the train to St Leonards, and then we walked quite some distance to the centre. As soon as I arrived, I met the centre's director and principal physiotherapist, Melissa McConaghy. Melissa is a neurological physiotherapist, and straight away she did an assessment of my condition.

Over the previous couple of years, Mum had been worrying that I had been walking better in Ballina Rehab than I was now, and she had been dwelling on Dr Cole's opinion that I would have a permanent limp. She was always hoping against hope that I would eventually walk well, whereas I was simply glad to be walking! Anyway, I passed the assessment with flying colours, so now Mum would have to eat her words.

'I think intensive rehab is for you,' Melissa said.

Melissa then gave all the details to Mum. Apparently the rehab would run for one month, and would involve a 'high volume of intervention', a 'multidisciplinary approach', and 'goal-directed therapy'. I wanted progress, and this sounded like the program for me!

Mum and I decided I would enter the program early the next year, after the summer holidays. I did that and it was intense. The staff there told me I could get results with my arm if I wanted to.

'The upper limb has potential,' they said.

I was ecstatic. I would give it a go. After all, what did I have to lose?

Every time I went to the Advance Rehab Centre I took a train instead of driving. All the days went from 9 am until 2.30 pm. By the end of each one, I was always exhausted.

I mainly worked with an occupational therapist called Lindsey who told me I would be going through the rehab program with another client – a man in his seventies, who had also had a stroke. The man's right arm was in a type of cast and he had a lovely smile. His wife was with him. They introduced themselves. They were Ron and Heather Causely.

Heather was a lot younger than Ron and was in great shape. She was really friendly and I liked her straight away. Ron could only say a few phrases. I felt sorry for him. Anyway, I became good friends with Ron and Heather. They lived in Sylvania, and right from that first day they offered to drive me home at the end of every day. This was such a blessing. I could catch the train to St Leonards every morning knowing I would get a ride home every afternoon!

The rehab was intensive and there was homework, too. I remember playing lots of computer games to help my right arm. A physiotherapist called Amanda Sleeman was in charge of these games. There was an apple game, and in the apple game a tree dropped apples and I had to catch them in the 'basket' on the screen by using my right hand to operate the joystick. As I played the game, the apples would drop faster and faster – and as I improved, I could increase the speed. There were other games as well, and they were all fun. Who knew I would have so much fun while working on my right arm?

Lindsey and Amanda were positive and encouraging. They identified several upper-limb tasks that I could do that involved my right hand, such as typing, grasping and releasing objects, tying a shoelace, using a knife and fork, and opening a door. I practised these things every day while I was there.

I also practised a marble task. Lindsey would give me marbles to help with my right hand. The task was to place the marbles in a basket with that hand by dropping them into it one by one. It was amazing how stuck I became with the release of the marbles! I would often curse at how difficult it was. Lindsey would also use playing cards and turn them upside down. My job was to turn them face-up just using my right hand. This was difficult as well but I didn't give up.

Meanwhile, part of my homework was to find a mirror and a shoebox. Lindsey wanted to make me a 'mirror box'. When I brought in the materials, she did this by cutting a hole in one of the small ends of the box, and then sticking the mirror along one of the long sides. She then asked me to place my right hand in the box, keeping it hidden from view, with the mirror facing my left hand. I would then have to make certain movements and perform little tasks with my left hand while watching its reflection in the mirror. As I did this, the reflection gave the illusion that it was actually my right hand! I know this therapy sounds complicated, but it was very effective and it did help trick my brain into believing my bad hand could do good things! It helped a lot.

Overall, attending the intensive rehabilitation program was a positive experience. The staff at the centre were wonderful. All the practice I was doing helped me improve both my walking and also the way I used my right hand. Heather was always around to encourage me, and one day she even took me to a lunchtime concert at the Sydney Conservatorium of Music. I felt that Ray was very lucky to have Heather, but Heather would always say she was lucky to have Ray. I could see why. Ray greeted me with a smile each day. I had made some more new friends!

So even though it had been annoying to fall over at the gallery and break my arm, the accident had led to something good. In the short term, I had taken one big step backwards in my recovery, but ultimately – because the accident had led me to the Advance Rehab Centre – I was now taking many more big steps forward.

Travel

Those steps have been so big they've taken me across the globe.

Thinking about this, I realise I have good associations with the name Meredith. Maybe this is because I not only have an aunt called Meredith, but also a friend with that name. And the crazy thing is that both women ended up with the same surname … but that's another story. For now, it's probably enough to say that I had Aunty Meredith, and a friend Meredith!

Anyway, I had been friends with Meredith for a few years but got to know her really well when we shared a little house together in Birchgrove. The house was right near the water. We had a lot of parties there. It was fun!

But Meredith wasn't only there for me in the good times. She was also a huge help to me after my stroke. I wanted to travel. I had always travelled with my family, and that's where my love for travel came from. Before my stroke, I had been to Europe and all over Australia. So in spite of my speech difficulties, I was determined to visit the places that inspired my imagination – both in Australia and overseas.

By this stage, Meredith was living in Port Douglas. I wanted to go to see her. I'd never been to Far North Queensland, but I'd always wanted to visit. This was my opportunity! I couldn't wait to breathe the balmy tropical air and swim in the warm sea.

I told my brother John this.

He said, 'Fantastic!'

But I sighed and explained that until my divorce was finalised, I couldn't afford the travel expenses. Then he offered to pay! So the long and the short of this was that I was going! I was very grateful to John, and also to my sister-in-law, Kirsty.

My trip started at Sydney Airport, where I caught a plane to Cairns. I then took a bus to Port Douglas. I collected my bag. Meredith had coached me on what to do next. She had said, 'You catch the bus and you say 20 Sand Street.'

I wondered what bus it would be. I was also worried about my speech but I thought it would be okay. Meredith said the bus ticket would be about $40 so I walked up to the official-looking counter and paying was easy, as I had the right money. I didn't have to count out any change. I walked out through the doors to the busy and bustling terminus.

A man in a blue uniform came up to me and said, 'Where are you going? This bus is to Cairns and this one to Port Douglas.'

I said, 'Port Douglas, please.' I hopped on a bus.

The scenery was just like I'd imagined – three-frond palm

trees and coconuts! I stared out the window, taking it all in. It was about sixty minutes to Port Douglas. Finally, I made it, and then we dropped people at hotels and hostels. I had some trouble explaining Meredith's address to the man. By that stage I was tired, and when I'm tired I have trouble speaking. But he eventually figured out what I was trying to say. Lucky for me Sand Street was well known; it was where a lot of tourists lived among the locals.

I got out. Meredith was there to greet me. She carried in the bag. I had arrived! I had made my first long solo trip since having the stroke. I was happy! So many times I'd told myself that I was determined to be well and capable again – and at last I felt that I had reached that goal.

The Travel Bug

But that first trip was only the first step. My trip to Port Douglas had strengthened my goal of recapturing as much of my old life as possible. These days, I am always dreaming about travelling.

Over the past ten years, I have been to many places. Recently, there was a ten-day cruise from Hong Kong to Singapore. And a few years before that, with my good friend Karen Riley, I travelled to Tasmania and the United States, including New York. While I liked New York, my favourite place was New Orleans. I loved New Orleans because the whole city was pulsating with jazz! At the Spotted Cat Jazz Club, I met the musician, Jamey St. Pierre and had a good chat with him.

Two women in the background were listening to the conversation. They overheard that I had had a stroke, and because they had a good friend who had also had a stroke, they complimented me on how brave I was to be out travelling across the world. Karen and I ended up having dinner with them!

I love these types of spontaneous experiences, which seem more likely to happen when I'm travelling. Not that travelling is easy! I still have a lot of trouble with stress and fatigue, and dealing with numbers can be confusing. While my maths is good, I struggle to convert currencies. And while I've always had a bad sense of direction, since having the stroke this is even worse. I've been lost all over the world!

Before my stroke I never had any difficulty speaking, but now I find that words won't come when I'm under stress … and this is more likely to happen when I'm travelling. I need to be calm for the words to come. I get tired easily when travelling and don't cope well with people being upset with me.

But I will keep travelling! It gives me a chance to learn about different cultures and see the way other people live. I feel elated when I travel. I love planning the trip and researching the destinations. Travel takes me out of my everyday life and gives me something to look forward to.

Next, I am determined to go on a 'Singing in Italy' trip with Stuart Davis. The trip will include visiting vineyards in Tuscany, listening to Gregorian chanting at the ancient San Miniato al Monte and singing with local choirs in Florence. Also, as Stuart promises, every day our travel group will form an 'instant choir' wherever it goes. After all, as Stuart likes to quote Ella Fitzgerald: 'The only thing better than singing is more singing.'

I couldn't agree more!

EPILOGUE

In the end it took three attempts to get the bulk carrier ship, the Pasha Bulker, back out to sea, and I guess you could say there was a similar pattern with me. I left Lismore Base Hospital, then Ballina Rehab, and finally the Advance Rehab Centre. Those were the three formal stages of my recovery.

Most people who know me understand how hard it was for me to make it through those stages. Rehabilitation specialist Dr Andrew Cole says most patients in my situation would have given up, while family members like Mum admire the way I always put a smile on my face and try my hardest. And then there are close friends like Jane who praise my 'optimistic spirit' and 'can-do attitude'. Jane calls me a 'champion'.

I don't feel like a champion. Yes, I do have a fighting spirit. But I didn't have a choice about having my stroke; it happened to me out of the blue. And since then, I just keep getting up on those mornings when I secretly don't want to, and I boost my spirits with singing. Overall, I simply try to stay determined in my efforts to improve. 'I will!' I tell myself out loud, over and over.

People like my parents are champions. My father was kind to everyone, and my mother has always been there for my youngest brother and me. Many times since my father and middle brother died I'm sure Mum has wanted to give up, but she never does. She keeps going and going. I don't know what I would do without her. She's a champion to me.

So are business owners like Bill Georgas, who after becoming a paraplegic began making driving aids for people with disabilities. And of course I will always see my brothers as champions – both Mark and John dedicated their careers to improving the lives of Indigenous Australians.

But me? I'm not a champion.

Maybe I'm more like Scout, the girl who tells the story about her father Atticus in *To Kill a Mockingbird* – the novel whose name I can now remember!

If you've ever read that book, you'll know that Scout is a go-getter, and she speaks from her heart. Most importantly, she learns from her father the importance of walking a mile in another person's shoes. Ultimately, Scout becomes the kind of person who makes herself and her family proud.

I think I will be happy with that.

JENNY'S SUGGESTIONS FOR STROKE SURVIVORS

Find Your Passion

If you have a passion, go with it. Singing is mine. I got well through singing. I don't know what would have happened if I hadn't been able to sing. I am forever grateful for that. I have belonged to many different choirs and am now singing with an *a cappella* group in Cronulla called the Sea Naturals. I enjoy it!

Never Give Up

I was told I would never be able to drive again but I was determined to get back behind the wheel. When I couldn't drive with a normal steering wheel, I learnt to drive my car using special driving aids. I didn't give up.

Be Grateful

No matter what your problems are, be positive and don't give in to your inner demons. I know you think this is easy for me to say, but even though I have been depressed about my situation (with no job, difficulty speaking and paralysis on the right side of my body), I still have so much to be grateful for (I'm walking, my left hand is working, and I enjoy life as much as I can). Ride through the rough times; you will be up again.

Relax

I don't know if you're the type of person who gets stressed out, but I was often stressed – especially over my work and my marriage. But I was very lucky to have my family and my friends, and also activities that make me feel calm: like swimming and singing. Meditation is also supposed to be a good thing to help you relax. I want to try it.

Use Your Brain

I did a TAFE course. Even though it was hard, it was the best thing I could have done. Not only did I end up with a formal qualification that has led to voluntary and paid work, but it also helped me to develop my speaking skills. It doesn't matter what the subject is – just follow your interests. I love Italy, so next I am going to do an Italian language course.

Volunteer

I do lots of volunteer work. This kind of work also takes me out of myself and stops me from thinking 'woe is me'. It shows me there are people much worse off than me and reminds me of how lucky I am. Volunteering gets me into a headspace of hope – hope that I can improve, and hope that I can be of service. If I go to an aged care centre and sing, for example, I might be feeling depressed on my way there, but then I see the looks on the residents' faces when we're all singing together, and it makes me happy!

Travel

I love to travel. Seeing different places gives me new perspectives on life. I can get to most places on my own, but prefer to travel with family, friends or a tour group. I find it difficult to talk when I'm under stress so it's best if I have someone with me at all times. If you're severely disabled and have no one to help you, don't lose hope. There are organisations such as Aspire Supported Holidays that can provide assisted holidays for travellers with disabilities or respite care requirements. Check out this wonderful organisation that my good friend Kate Somerville told me about: www.aspiresupportedholidays.com.au/

Medication

Drugs like anti-depressants can be lifesavers. If you get depressed after a stroke they can really help, especially when every little bit of help counts. Don't be afraid to take them if you need to. They helped me get out of a really dark place.

Nurturing Friends

Friends come and go. Some fall by the wayside; don't worry about that. Others surprise you by going above and beyond what you ever expect. Also, make new friends. I make new friends all the time. When I worked as a teacher, it was easy to make friends in my workplace, but I lost that part of my life. So I joined social groups like choirs and art therapy groups, and despite my disability I made friends. I wasn't able to talk a lot but when I said 'stroke' people understood. I am now talking so well that most people don't realise I've had a stroke. Friends can be there to listen and support you in so many ways, just as you can be there for them. I don't know what I'd do without my friends.

Seek Counselling

At the end of my marriage I looked around for a counsellor. I found an excellent one and I have been seeing her for nearly a decade. I tell her things I wouldn't tell anyone else. She helped put the end of my marriage into perspective. Leaving my marriage was the hardest thing to do but she helped me understand that it was a toxic relationship, and that it was far better for me to leave than stay. With her help, I'm so much better off now. I'm single and am living life to the fullest. Fortunately, I found an instant rapport with my counsellor. If you're not getting anything from your counsellor, look around for someone else. Trust that you will eventually find a counsellor who is on your wavelength.

Live Healthy

Health is important. I had a stroke so I take particular care with my health, as I don't want to have another one. I have a healthy diet that includes lots of vegetables, and I walk every day and I go to the gym. I have a trainer. She became a friend. As well as keeping me fit, the gym helps me de-stress. I'm also glad I can walk to the gym; it's nice to take a walk on a sunny day. There is nothing that compares!

Catch Some Sun – With Protection

Try to get out in the sun. There's nothing like those rays. The safest time of the day to do this is mid-morning or mid-afternoon, and only for about ten or fifteen minutes. Being in the sunshine can help with depression, and it also helps your body create Vitamin D. When I worked at an aged care centre, I tried to get the residents in regency chairs out in the sunshine. They loved this!

Acupuncture Helps

I had a boyfriend once who was training to be an acupuncturist. I wasn't frightened of needles so I volunteered as the 'guinea pig'. I did this a lot of times and it helped me. When I moved back to Sydney I found a qualified acupuncturist. This therapy improves things for me in mental, emotional and physical ways. If you're afraid of needles it won't do for you, but if you're not afraid give it a try!

Try Advanced Rehab

Improve your daily living skills, health and wellbeing by going to a centre where you can complete an intensive rehabilitation program. I went to Advance Care Rehab in St Leonards and it was like going to a stroke survivor boot camp every day! I worked hard there, and the program not only improved my walking but also helped me get more use out of my damaged hand.

Attempt New Things … and Do Old Things Differently

I used to do things without thought, like talking, chopping tomatoes, cutting paper with scissors and putting on a bra. After my stroke I had to learn these things all over again – mostly in different ways. I felt like I was stuck in a nightmare, but I was determined to get better. With the help of occupational therapists, I learnt different ways to get things done. Some of the new ways have turned out to be good!

Trust That Life Will Improve

As Scarlet O'Hara says in *Gone with the Wind*, 'Tomorrow is another day.' Try to think of that! I know what it is to be in the depths of despair with no easy way out, feeling hopeless and alone. But the very next day help can come along or something lovely can happen. Try to get help and be positive. After all, there is only one you in the world.

Helpful Contacts

> Stroke Foundation (an organisation dedicated to stroke recovery and support)
> 1800 787 653
> https://strokefoundation.org.au/
>
> Lifeline (24-hour phone counselling service)
> 13 11 95
> https://www.lifeline.org.au/
>
> Beyond Blue (for help with depression)
> 1300 244 636
> www.beyondblue.org.au
>
> Black Dog Institute (for help with depression)
> 9382 4505
> www.blackdoginstitute.org.au

FROM THE SAME PUBLISHER

A Taste for Diamonds

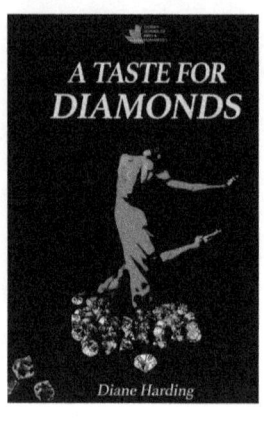

A diamond theft. A fateful dancer. Passion, love and money in a story that unfolds through the rhythm of the tango.

'A Taste for Diamonds' is a love story that spans two continents, from London to Buenos Aires, as Harriett and the man she loves – the man who loves her in return – face the consequences of getting involved in the international diamond trade.

Not everyone's a good guy, as they find out to their peril.

Author **Diane Harding** plumbs the depths of romance and intrigue to bring readers a satisfying ending to a dangerous tale of love.

Category: BOOKS – MYSTERY – THRILLER – CRIME

An extraordinary relationship

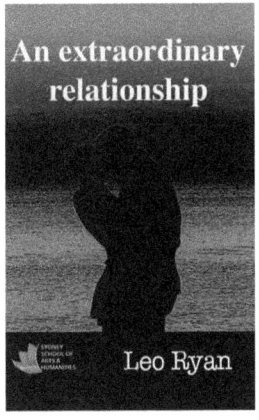

Early in **Leo Ryan**'s career as a counsellor he became aware of the number of female clients being abused by their husbands/ partners/boyfriends and was determined to help.

This book highlights his conclusions, making it possible for most people to bring on the changes needed have a great relationship.

Category: NON-FICTION – HOW-TO BOOK
RELATIONSHIPS

Burma My Mother
And Why I Had To Leave

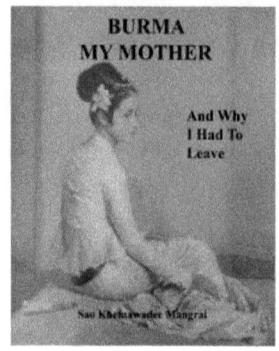

Myanmar's future is informed by its past - and BURMA MY MOTHER tells it like it is.

A valuable story of living through good times and plenty of bad in Burma, now known as Myanmar, before an escape to a new life of freedom.

Author **Sao Khemawadee Mangrai**'s husband, Hom, was imprisoned for 5 years, and his father was shot and killed sitting alongside independence leader, General Aung San, when he was assassinated.

Khemawadee grew up in a Shan state in the north-east of Myanmar, previously known as Burma, and now lives in Sydney. Her sad memories are also infused by the beauty of the country and the grace of Myanmar's Buddhist culture.

Category: MEMOIR

Drenched by the Sun

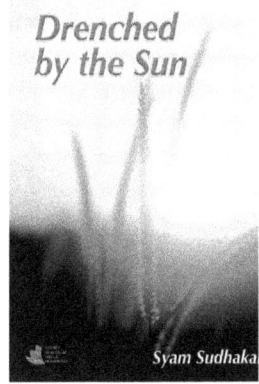

**I, who prophesy
by reading the stars and the wind,
now think of that country ...**

Syam Sudhakar 'has an eye for the strange and the uncanny and a way of building translucent metaphors,' according to leading South Indian poet, K. Satchidanandan.

An award-winning poet who writes in English and Malayalam, Sudhakar is based in Kerala, teaching and researching Indian poetry.

Category: POEMS

Night Road to Life

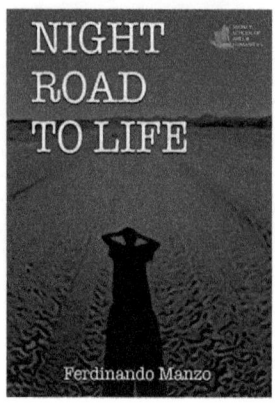

Themes of the sea and the emotions, particularly the deeply felt joys and melancholies experienced by men, are a touchstone of NIGHT ROAD TO LIFE.

Ferdinando Manzo's thoughts are not bound to fluidity; they fly to the greatest heights of exhilaration in poems such as, *The sky above us*, which displays 'a mantle of stars that burns in my heart' and in the evocative lines of *Eclipse*: 'the moon rose, bright between the eyelids of the night'.

Even the constellation Andromeda is given due recognition, breaking her chains and ready for revenge, before another poem *The voice of the universe* explores 'a hidden legend as far away as waves in outer space'.

A distinctive quality of this collection of poems is its musicality – the sounds of words carefully chosen, and their rhythms. The pleasing effect of the sensuality of sounds, ranging from gentleness to the drama of sex, is in tune with the gamut of human emotion.

Category: POEMS

Reported Missing

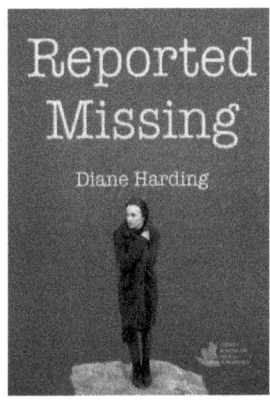

Di Harding's novel is set in a very contemporary Sydney, taking in multi-layered sights and sounds, from the northern beaches to performances at the Sydney Opera House.

The plot spans the complications of what a woman must consider if she is to save her children from domestic violence. And the main character has good reason to hold fears for her life.

What would you do if your daughter was missing and you thought your son-in-law was somehow involved? Is there someone who could help you, or would you take matters into your own hands?

She does, and so the terror begins – from vile and personal harassment to life threatening acts, until she is ready to commit murder.

Her obsession with killing grows in her mind until she begins to plan and plot. Can she actually do it? Then something shocking happens to make up her mind.

The story ends on an upbeat for a new life ahead for the family.

Category: DOMESTIC VIOLENCE
           CRIME FICTION – SYDNEY NOVEL
           AUSTRALIAN FICTION

Road to Mandalay Less Travelled

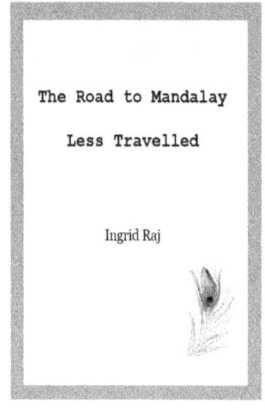

'The Road to Mandalay Less Travelled' by **Ingrid Raj** provides research on a selection of Anglo-Burmese writing published from the period of British rule in Burma up until 2007.

What Raj shares with us in this study is the knowledge she gained about the value of social resistance achieved through writing. Both fiction and non-fiction texts are included in arguing a case that these might be viewed as tools of often ambivalent resistance against oppressive regimes, both local and colonial. Her research deserves a wider readership than was initially provided, and to this aim Sydney School of Arts & Humanities presents the work as its first publication in this new category of Essays & Theses.

We hope that specialist researchers as well as members of the general reading public take this opportunity to learn more about the culture of the people of Myanmar through their unique approach to storytelling, based largely on their religious understanding, their rich store of folk legend and their chequered history.

Category: MEMOIR – LITERATURE – BURMA – HISTORY

Road to Rishi Konda

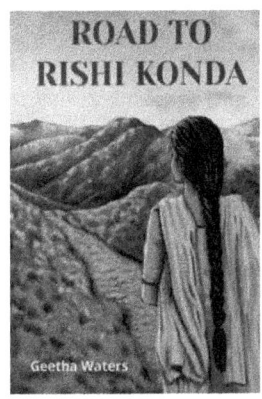

'ROAD TO RISHI KONDA' by **Geetha Waters** is a memoir of insight and charm, with a serious educational purpose. The author recalls delightful and stimulating stories from her childhood to throw light on the work of the philosopher J. Krishnamurti as a revolutionary 20th century educator.

At once fascinating and enchanting, Geetha Waters' stories centre on a girl growing up in Kerala and Andhra Pradesh in the '60s and '70s.

These youthful tales are underpinned by Geetha's deep understanding of childhood education, based both on her academic studies and in practice in her daily life as a mother and childcare professional.

Written from a child's perspective, the tales of awakening to life offer the reader an opportunity to appreciate how all children learn, as they draw on a deep well of curiosity that needs to be respected.

Category: BIOGRAPHY & AUTOBIOGRAPHY
PERSONAL MEMOIR – EDUCATORS

Stranger

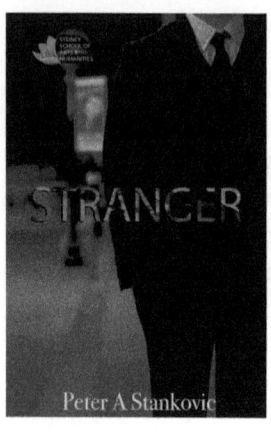

Political journalist Nick Hunter suddenly loses his memory. He can't find his wallet, his computer password or even his name. When it comes to women it's even more confusing. Does he have a lover or a wife?

It doesn't get any easier when he realises his life is in danger as he's been researching a story on corruption at the highest level of political life. Things get even stickier once Nick has a 6-shooter out of his safety deposit box and in his hand, ready to fire in his own defence.

Set in the northern and eastern suburbs of Sydney where coffee and sex are almost too freely available, this story will sharpen your senses and set your crime thriller compass on true course.

Category: FICTION – CRIME

The Dark Side of the Opera

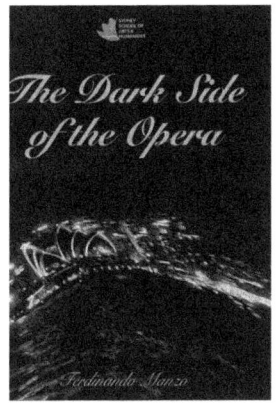

In this collection, **Ferdinando Manzo** plays with language, teasing out meaning and tempting the senses. His poetic approach is akin to the Buddhist path where happiness is gained through an understanding of negation.

From the earthly to the stellar, each poem holds the reader in suspense until the final moment.

Category: POEMS

Waking the Mind

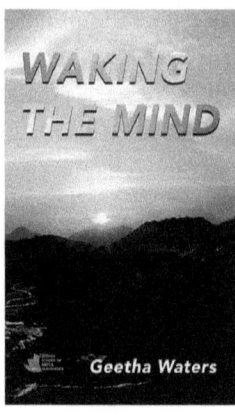

Geetha Waters' engaging selection of short stories, 'Waking the Mind', is a reflection on Jiddu Krishnamurti's impact on her education based on her experiences at a school he founded in South India.

Geetha credits her passion for inquiry as being sparked the first time she heard Krishnamurti speak when she was six. That talk at the Rishi Valley School set her on an intriguing course of inquiry into the mysterious nature of the mind, the vitality of the natural world, and a creative understanding of life.

'Waking the Mind' is Geetha Waters' second book, following 'Road to Rishi Konda', her stories of a girl growing up in Kerala and Andhra Pradesh in the '60s and '70s.

Geetha Waters also incorporates the stories found in 'Road to Rishi Konda' in the STEP program for children and teachers in South India, a training module based on Krishnamurti's interactive style of relating with children.

Category: NON-FICTION – INDIAN STORIES – PHILOSOPHY
KRISHNAMURTI

What's in a Name?
20 People - 20 Stories

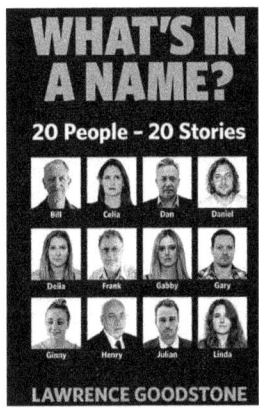

This collection of short stories will appeal to readers who are attracted to snapshots of the human condition. While set in Australia, the stories reflect universal themes. They range over a number of genres from crime to science fiction, from human weakness to human strength, and capture pockets of life with uncanny accuracy and sensitivity.

The author, **Lawrence Goodstone**, is a retired public servant who spent his professional life writing for others. With a background ranging from teaching to immigrant services as well as assisting in the delivery of the 2000 Olympic Games in Sydney, he is now in a position to write for himself and create stories from a life well lived.

Category: FICTION – SHORT STORY – SYDNEY STORIES
AUSTRALIAN FICTION

Jiddu Krishnamurti World Philosopher
Revised Edition

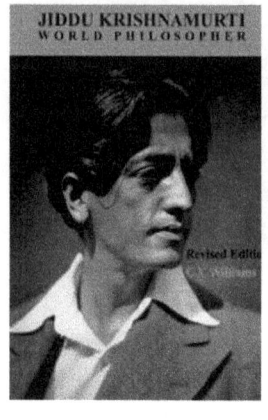

The life of the 20th-century philosopher Jiddu Krishnamurti was truly astonishing. As this new updated edition shows, people from all over the world would gather to hear him speak the wisdom of the ages.

Biographer **Christine (CV) Williams** carried out research over a period of four years to write this ebook account of Krishnamurti's life. She studied his major archive of personal correspondence and talks, and interviewed people who knew him intimately.

Krishna was born into poverty in a South Indian village, before being adopted by a wealthy English public figure, Annie Besant. As an adult he settled in California, travelling to India and England every year to give public lectures that inspired spiritual seekers beyond any single religion.

Category: BIOGRAPHY

www.ingramcontent.com/pod-product-compliance
Lightning Source LLC
Chambersburg PA
CBHW032119040426
42449CB00005B/195